Human Foods and Their Nutritive Value

By Harry Snyder

PREFACE

Since 1897 instruction has been given at the University of Minnesota, College of Agriculture, on human foods and their nutritive value. With the development of the work, need has been felt for a text-book presenting in concise form the composition and physical properties of foods, and discussing some of the main factors which affect their nutritive value. To meet the need, this book has been prepared, primarily for the author's classroom. It aims to present some of the principles of human nutrition along with a study of the more common articles of food. It is believed that a better understanding of the subject of nutrition will suggest ways in which foods may be selected and utilized more intelligently, resulting not only in pecuniary saving, but also in greater efficiency of physical and mental effort.

Prominence is given in this work to those foods, as flour, bread, cereals, vegetables, meats, milk, dairy products, and fruits, that are most extensively used in the dietary, and to some of the physical, chemical, and bacteriological changes affecting digestibility and nutritive value which take place during their preparation for the table. Dietary studies, comparative cost and value of foods, rational feeding of men, and experiments and laboratory practice form features of the work. Some closely related topics, largely of a sanitary nature, as the effect upon food of household sanitation and storage, are also briefly discussed. References are given in case more extended information is desired on some of the subjects treated. While this book was prepared mainly for students who have taken a course in general chemistry, it has been the intention to present the topics in such a way as to be understood by the layman also.

This work completes a series of text-books undertaken by the author over ten years ago, dealing with agricultural and industrial subjects: "Chemistry of Plant and Animal Life," "Dairy Chemistry," "Soils and Fertilizers," and "Human Foods and their Nutritive Value." It has been the aim in preparing these books to avoid as far as possible repetition, but at the same time to make each work sufficiently complete to permit its use as a text independent of the series.

One of the greatest uses that science can serve is in its application to the household and the everyday affairs of life. Too little attention is generally bestowed upon the study of foods in schools and colleges, and the author sincerely hopes the time will soon come when more prominence will be given to this subject, which is the oldest, most important, most neglected, and least understood of any that have a direct bearing upon the welfare of man.

HARRY SNYDER.

CONTENTS

CHAPTER I

CHAPTER II

CHANGES IN COMPOSITION OF FOODS DURING COOKING AND PREPARATION

CHAPTER VI

LEGUMES AND NUTS

General Composition of Legumes; Beans; Digestibility of Beans; Use of Beans in the Dietary; String Beans; Peas; Canned Peas; Peanuts; General Composition of Nuts; Chestnuts; The Hickory Nut; Almonds; Pistachio; Cocoanuts; Uses of Nuts in the Dietary.

CHAPTER VII

MILK AND DAIRY PRODUCTS

Importance in the Dietary; General Composition; Digestibility; Sanitary Condition of Milk; Certified Milk; Pasteurized Milk; Tyrotoxicon; Color of Milk; Souring of Milk; Use of Preservatives in Milk; Condensed Milk; Skim Milk; Cream; Buttermilk; Goat's Milk; Koumiss; Prepared Milks; Human Milk; Adulteration of Milk; Composition of Butter; Digestibility of Butter; Adulteration of Butter; General Composition of Cheese; Digestibility; Use in the Dietary; Cottage Cheese; Different Kinds of Cheese; Adulteration of Cheese; Dairy Products in the Dietary.

CHAPTER VIII

MEATS AND ANIMAL FOOD PRODUCTS

General Composition; Mineral Matter; Fat; Protein; Non-nitrogenous Compounds; Why Meats vary in Composition; Amides; Albuminoids; Taste and Flavor of Meats; Alkaloidal Bodies in Meats; Ripening of Meats in Cold Storage; Beef; Veal; Mutton; Pork; Lard; Texture and Toughness of Meat; Influence of Cooking upon the Composition of Meats; Beef Extracts; Miscellaneous Meat Products; Pickled Meats; Saltpeter in Meats; Smoked Meats; Poultry; Fish; Oysters, Fattening of; Shell Fish; Eggs, General Composition; Digestibility of Eggs; Use of Eggs in the Dietary; Canned

Meats, General Composition.

CHAPTER IX

CEREALS

Preparation and Cost of Cereals; Various Grains used in making Cereal Products; Cleanliness of; Corn Preparations; Corn Flour; Use of Corn in Dietary; Corn Bread; Oat Preparations; Cooking of Oatmeal; Wheat Preparations; Flour Middlings; Breakfast Foods; Digestibility of Wheat Preparations; Barley Preparations; Rice Preparations; Predigested Foods; The Value of Cereals in the Dietary; Phosphate Content of Cereals; Phosphorus Requirements of a Ration; Mechanical Action of Cereals upon Digestion; Cost and Nutritive Value of Cereals.

CHAPTER X

WHEAT FLOUR

Use for Bread Making; Winter and Spring Wheat Flours; Composition of Wheat and Flour; Roller Process of Flour Milling; Grades of Flour; Types of Flour; Composition of Flour; Graham and Entire Wheat Flours; Composition of Wheat Offals; Aging and Curing of Flour; Macaroni Flour; Color; Granulation; Capacity of Flour to absorb Water; Physical Properties of Gluten; Gluten as a Factor in Bread Making; Unsoundness; Comparative Baking Tests; Bleaching; Adulteration of Flour; Nutritive Value of Flour.

CHAPTER XI

BREAD AND BREAD MAKING

Leavened and Unleavened Bread; Changes during Bread Making; Loss of Dry Matter during Bread Making; Action of Yeast; Compressed Yeast; Dry Yeast; Production of Carbon Dioxid Gas and Alcohol; Production of Soluble

Carbohydrates; Production of Acids in Bread Making; Volatile Compounds produced during Bread Making; Behavior of Wheat Proteids in Bread Making; Production of Volatile Nitrogenous Compounds; Oxidation of Fat; Influence of the Addition of Wheat Starch and Gluten to Flour; Composition of Bread; Use of Skim Milk and Lard in Bread Making; Influence of Warm and Cold Flours in Bread Making; Variations in the Process of Bread Making; Digestibility of Bread; Use of Graham and Entire Wheat in the Dietary; Mineral Content of White Bread; Comparative Digestibility of New and Old Bread; Different Kinds of Bread; Toast.

CHAPTER XII

BAKING POWDERS

General Composition; Cream of Tartar Powders; Residue from Cream of Tartar Baking Powders; Tartaric Acid Powders; Phosphate Baking Powders; Mineral and Organic Phosphates; Phosphate Residue; Alum Baking Powders; Residue from Alum Baking Powders; Objections urged against Alum Powders; Action of Baking Powders and Yeast Compared; Keeping Qualities of Baking Powders; Inspection of Baking Powders; Fillers; Home-made Baking Powders.

CHAPTER XIII

VINEGAR, SPICES, AND CONDIMENTS

Vinegar; Chemical Changes during Manufacture of Vinegar; Ferment Action; Materials used in Preparation of Vinegars; Characteristics of a Good Vinegar; Vinegar Solids; Acidity of Vinegar; Different Kinds of Vinegars; Standards of Purity; Adulteration of Vinegar; Characteristics of Spices; Pepper; Cayenne; Mustard; Ginger; Cinnamon and Cassia; Cloves; Allspice; Nutmeg; Adulteration of Spices and Condiments; Essential Oils of; Uses of Condiments in Preparation of Foods; Action of Condiments upon Digestion; Condiments and Natural Flavors.

CHAPTER XVII

DIETARY STUDIES

Object of Dietary Studies; Wide and Narrow Rations; Dietary Standards; Number of Meals per Day; Mixed Dietary Desirable; Animal and Vegetable Foods; Economy of Production; Food Habits; Underfed Families; Cheap and Expensive Foods; Food Notions; Dietary of Two Families Compared; Food in its Relation to Mental and Physical Vigor; Dietary Studies in Public Institutions.

CHAPTER XVIII

RATIONAL FEELING OF MAN

Object; Human and Animal Feeding Compared; Standard Rations; Why Tentative Dietary Standards; Amounts of Food Consumed; Average Composition of Foods; Variations in Composition of Foods; Example of a Ration; Calculations of Balanced Rations; Requisites of a Balanced Ration; Examples; Calculations of Rations for Men at Different Kinds of Labor.

CHAPTER XIX

WATER

Importance; Impurities in Water; Mineral Impurities; Organic Impurities; Interpretation of a Water Analysis; Natural Purification of Water; Water in Relation to Health; Improvement of Waters; Boiling of Water; Filtration; Purification of Water by Addition of Chemicals; Ice; Rain Waters; Waters of High and Low Purity; Chemical Changes which Organic Matter of Water Undergoes; Bacterial Content of Water; Mineral Waters; Materials for Softening Water; Uses of; Economic Value of a Pure Water Supply.

CHAPTER XX

FOOD AS AFFECTED BY HOUSEHOLD SANITATION AND STORAGE

Injurious Compounds in Foods; Nutrient Content and Sanitary Condition of Food; Sources of Contamination of Food; Unclean Ways of Handling Food; Sanitary Inspection of Food; Infection from Impure Air; Storage of Food in Cellars; Respiration of Vegetable Cells; Sunlight, Pure Water, and Pure Air as Disinfectants; Foods contaminated from Leaky Plumbing; Utensils for Storage of Food; Contamination from Unclean Dishcloths; Refrigeration; Chemical Changes that take Place in the Refrigerator; Soil; Disposal of Kitchen Refuse; Germ Diseases spread by Unsanitary Conditions around Dwellings due to Contamination of Food; General Considerations; Relation of Food to Health.

CHAPTER XXI

LABORATORY PRACTICE

Object of Laboratory Practice; Laboratory Note-book and Suggestions for Laboratory Practice; List of Apparatus Used; Photograph of Apparatus Used; Directions for Weighing; Directions for Measuring; Use of Microscope; Water in Flour; Water in Butter; Ash in Flour; Nitric Acid Test for Nitrogenous Organic Matter; Acidity of Lemons; Influence of Heat on Potato Starch Grains; Influence of Yeast on Starch Grains; Mechanical Composition of Potatoes; Pectose from Apples; Lemon Extract; Vanilla Extract; Testing Olive Oil for Cotton Seed Oil; Testing for Coal Tar Dyes; Determining the Per Cent of Skin in Beans; Extraction of Fat from Peanuts; Microscopic Examination of Milk; Formaldehyde in Cream or Milk; Gelatine in Cream or Milk; Testing for Oleomargarine; Testing for Watering or Skimming of Milk; Boric Acid in Meat; Microscopic Examination of Cereal Starch Grains; Identification of Commercial Cereals; Granulation and Color of Flour; Capacity of Flour to absorb Water; Acidity of Flour; Moist and Dry Gluten; Gliadin from Flour; Bread-making Test; Microscopic Examination of Yeast; Testing Baking Powders for Alum; Testing Baking Powders for Phosphoric Acid; Testing Baking Powders for Ammonia; Vinegar Solids; Specific Gravity of Vinegar; Acidity of Vinegar; Deportment of Vinegar with Reagents; Testing Mustard for Turmeric; Examination of Tea Leaves; Action of Iron Compounds upon Tannic Acid; Identification of Coffee Berries; Detecting Chicory in Coffee; Comparative Amounts of Soap Necessary with Hard and Soft Water; Solvent Action of Water on Lead; Suspended Matter in Water; Organic Matter in Water; Deposition of Lime by Boiling Water; Qualitative Tests for Minerals in Water; Testing for Nitrites in Water.

REVIEW QUESTIONS

CHAPTER I

GENERAL COMPOSITION OF FOODS

1. Water.--All foods contain water. Vegetables in their natural condition contain large amounts, often 95 per cent, while in meats there is from 40 to 60 per cent or more. Prepared cereal products, as flour, corn meal, and oatmeal, which are apparently dry, have from 7 to 14 per cent. In general the amount of water in a food varies with the mechanical structure and the conditions under which it has been prepared, and is an important factor in estimating the value, as the nutrients are often greatly decreased because of large amounts of water. The water in substances as flour and meal is mechanically held in combination with the fine particles and varies with the moisture content, or hydroscopicity, of the air. Oftentimes foods gain or lose water to such an extent as to affect their weight; for example, one hundred pounds of flour containing 12 per cent of water may be reduced in weight three pounds or more when stored in a dry place, or there may be an increase in weight from being stored in a damp place. In tables of analyses the results, unless otherwise stated, are usually given on the basis of the original material, or the dry substance. Potatoes, for example, contain 2-1/2 per cent of crude protein on the basis of 75 per cent of water; or on a dry matter basis, that is, when the water is entirely eliminated, there is 10 per cent of protein.

The water of foods is determined by drying the weighed material in a water or air oven at a temperature of about 100?C, until all of the moisture has been expelled in the form of steam, leaving the dry matter or material free from water.[1] The determination of dry matter, while theoretically a simple process, is attended with many difficulties. Substances which contain much fat may undergo oxidation during drying; volatile compounds, as essential oils, are expelled along with the moisture; and other changes may occur affecting the accuracy of the work. The last traces of moisture are removed with difficulty from a substance, being mechanically retained by the particles with great tenacity. When very accurate dry matter determinations are desired, the substance is dried in a vacuum oven, or in a desiccator over sulphuric acid, or in an atmosphere of some non-oxidizing gas, as hydrogen.

2. Dry Matter.--The dry matter of a food is a mechanical mixture of the various compounds, as starch, sugar, fat, protein, cellulose, and mineral matter, and is obtained by drying the material. Succulent vegetable foods with 95 per cent of water contain only 5 per cent of dry matter, while in flour with 12 per cent of water there is 88 per cent, and in sugar 99 per cent. The dry matter is obtained by subtracting the per cent of water from 100, and in foods it varies from 5 per cent and less in some vegetables to 99 per cent in sugar.

1, desiccator; 2, muffle furnace for combustion of foods and obtaining ash; 3, water oven for drying food materials.]

3. Ash.--The ash, or mineral matter, is that portion obtained by burning or igniting the dry matter at the lowest temperature necessary for complete combustion. The ash in vegetable foods ranges from 2 to 5 per cent and, together with the nitrogen, represents what was taken from the soil during growth. In animal bodies, the ash is present mainly in the bones, but there is also an appreciable amount, one per cent or more, in all the tissues. Ash is exceedingly variable in composition, being composed of the various salts of potassium, sodium, calcium, magnesium, and iron, as sulphates, phosphates, chlorides, and silicates of these elements. There are also other elements in small amounts. In the plant economy these elements take an essential part and are requisite for the formation of plant tissue and the production in the leaves of the organic compounds which later are stored up in the seeds. Some of the elements appear to be more necessary than others, and whenever withheld plant growth is restricted. The elements most essential for plant growth are potassium, calcium, magnesium, iron, phosphorus, and sulphur.[1]

In the animal body minerals are derived, either directly or indirectly, from the vegetable foods consumed. The part which each of the mineral elements takes in animal nutrition is not well understood. Some of the elements, as phosphorus and sulphur, are in organic combination with the nitrogenous compounds, as the nucleated albuminoids, which are very essential for animal life. In both plant and animal bodies, the mineral matter is present as mineral salts and organic combinations. It is held that the ash elements which are in organic combination are the forms mainly utilized for tissue construction. While it is not known just what part all the mineral elements take in animal nutrition, experiments show that in all ordinary mixed rations the amount of the different mineral elements is in excess of the demands of the body, and it is only in rare instances, as in cases of restricted diet, or convalescence from some disease, that special attention need be given to increasing the mineral content of the ration. An excess of mineral matter in foods is equally as objectionable as a scant amount, elimination of the excess entailing additional work on the body.

The composition of the ash of different food materials varies widely, both in amount, and form of the individual elements. When for any reason it is necessary to increase the phosphates in a ration, milk and eggs do this to a greater extent than almost any other foods. Common salt, or sodium chloride, is one of the most essential of the mineral constituents of the body. It is necessary for giving the blood its normal composition, furnishing acid and basic constituents for the production of the digestive fluids, and for the nutrition of the cells. While salt is a necessary food, in large amounts, as when the attempt is made to use sea water as a beverage, it acts as a poison, suggesting that a material may be both a food and a poison. When sodium chloride is entirely withheld from an animal, death from salt starvation ensues. Many foods contain naturally small amounts of sodium chloride.

4. Organic Matter.--That portion of a food material which is converted into gaseous or volatile products during combustion is called the organic matter. It is a mechanical mixture of compounds made up of carbon, hydrogen, oxygen, nitrogen, and sulphur, and is composed of various individual organic compounds, as cellulose, starch, sugar, albumin, and fat. The

amount in a food is determined by subtracting the ash and water from 100. The organic matter varies widely in composition; in some foods it is largely starch, as in potatoes and rice, while in others, as forage crops consumed by animals, cellulose predominates. The nature of the prevailing organic compound, as sugar or starch, determines the nutritive value of a food. Each has a definite chemical composition capable of being expressed by a formula. Considered collectively, the organic compounds are termed organic matter. When burned, the organic compounds are converted into gases, the carbon uniting with the oxygen of the air to form carbon dioxide, hydrogen to form water, sulphur to form sulphur dioxide, and the nitrogen to form oxides of nitrogen and ammonia.

5. Classification of Organic Compounds.--All food materials are composed of a large number of organic compounds. For purposes of study these are divided into classes. The element nitrogen is taken as the basis of the division. Compounds which contain this element are called nitrogenous, while those from which it is absent are called non-nitrogenous.[2] The nitrogenous organic compounds are composed of the elements nitrogen, hydrogen, carbon, oxygen, and sulphur, while the non-nitrogenous compounds are composed of carbon, hydrogen, and oxygen. In vegetable foods the non-nitrogenous compounds predominate, there being usually from six to twelve parts of non-nitrogenous to every one part of nitrogenous, while in animal foods the nitrogenous compounds are present in larger amount.

NON-NITROGENOUS COMPOUNDS

6. Occurrence.--The non-nitrogenous compounds of foods consist mainly of cellulose, starch, sugar, and fat. For purposes of study, they are divided into subdivisions, as carbohydrates, pectose substances or jellies, fats, organic acids, essential oils, and mixed compounds. In plants the carbohydrates predominate, while in animal tissue the fats are the chief non-nitrogenous constituents.

7. Carbohydrates.--This term is applied to a class of compounds similar in general composition, but differing widely in structural composition and physical properties. Carbohydrates make up the bulk of vegetable foods and, except in milk, are found only in traces in animal foods. They are all represented by the general formula $CH_{2n}2n$, there being twice as many hydrogen as oxygen atoms, the hydrogen and oxygen being present in the same proportion as in water. As a class, the carbohydrates are neutral bodies, and, when burned, form carbon dioxide and water.

8. Cellulose is the basis of the cell structure of plants, and is found in various physical forms in food materials.[3] Sometimes it is hard and dense, resisting digestive action and mechanically inclosing other nutrients and thus preventing their being available as food. In the earlier stages of plant growth a part of the cellulose is in chemical combination with water, forming hydrated cellulose, a portion of which undergoes digestion and produces heat and energy in the body. Ordinarily, however, cellulose adds but little in the way of nutritive value, although it is often beneficial mechanically and imparts bulk to some foods otherwise too concentrated. The mechanical action of cellulose on the digestion of food is discussed in Chapter XV. Cellulose usually makes up a very small part of human food, less than 1 per cent. In refined white flour there is less than .05 of a per cent; in oatmeal and cereal products from .5 to 1 per cent, depending upon the extent to which the hulls are removed, and in vegetable foods from .1 to 1 per cent. The cellulose content of foods is included in the crude fiber of the chemist's report.

9. Starch occurs widely distributed in nature, particularly in the seeds, roots, and tubers of some plants. It is formed in the leaves of plants as a result of the joint action of chlorophyll and protoplasm, and is generally held by plant physiologists to be the first carbohydrate produced in the plant cell. Starch is composed of a number of overlapping layers separated by starch cellulose; between these layers the true starch or amylose is found. Starch from the various cereals and vegetables differs widely in mechanical structure; in wheat it is circular, in corn somewhat angular, and in parsnips exceedingly

small, while potato starch granules are among the largest.[4] The nature of starch can be determined largely from its mechanical structure as studied under the microscope. It is insoluble in cold water because of the protecting action of the cellular layer, but on being heated it undergoes both mechanical and chemical changes; the grains are partially ruptured by pressure due to the conversion into steam of the moisture held mechanically. The cooking of foods is beneficial from a mechanical point of view, as it results in partial disintegration of the starch masses, changing the structure so that the starch is more readily acted upon by the ferments of the digestive tract. At a temperature of about 120?C. starch begins to undergo chemical change, resulting in the rearrangement of the atoms in the molecule with the production of dextrine and soluble carbohydrates. Dextrine is formed on the crust of bread, or whenever potatoes or starchy foods are browned. At a still higher temperature starch is decomposed, with the liberation of water and production of compounds of higher carbon content. When heated in contact with water, it undergoes hydration changes; gelatinous-like products are formed, which are finally converted into a soluble condition. In cooking cereals, the hydration of the starch is one of the main physical and chemical changes that takes place, and it simply results in converting the material into such a form that other chemical changes may more readily occur. Before starch becomes dextrose, hydration is necessary. If this is accomplished by cooking, it saves the body just so much energy in digestion. Many foods owe their value largely to the starch. In cereals it is found to the extent of 72 to 76 per cent; in rice and potatoes in still larger amounts; and it is the chief constituent of many vegetables. When starch is digested, it is first changed to a soluble form and then gradually undergoes oxidation, resulting in the production of heat and energy, the same products--carbon dioxide and water--being formed as when starch is burned. Starch is a valuable heat-producing nutrient; a pound yields 1860 calories. See Chapter XV.

10. Sugar.--Sugars are widely distributed in nature, being found principally in the juices of the sugar cane, sugar beet, and sugar maple. They are divided into two large classes: the sucrose group and the dextrose group, the latter being produced from sucrose, starch, and other carbohydrates by inversion

and allied chemical changes. Because of the importance of sugar in the dietary, Chapter V is devoted to the subject.

11. Pectose Substances are jelly-like bodies found in fruits and vegetables. They are closely related in chemical composition to the carbohydrates, into which form they are changed during digestion; and in nutrition they serve practically the same function. In the early stages of growth the pectin bodies are combined with organic acids, forming insoluble compounds, as the pectin in green apples. During the ripening of fruit and the cooking of vegetables, the pectin is changed to a more soluble and digestible condition. In food analysis, the pectin is usually included with the carbohydrates.

12. Nitrogen-free-extract.--In discussing the composition of foods, the carbohydrates other then cellulose, as starch, sugar, and pectin, are grouped under the name of nitrogen-free-extract. Methods of chemical analysis have not yet been sufficiently perfected to enable accurate and rapid determination to be made of all these individual carbohydrates, and hence they are grouped together as nitrogen-free-extract. As the name indicates, they are compounds which contain no nitrogen, and are extractives in the sense that they are soluble in dilute acid and alkaline solutions. The nitrogen-free-extract is determined indirectly, that is, by the method of difference. All the other constituents of a food, as water, ash, crude fiber (cellulose), crude protein, and ether extract, are determined; the total is subtracted from 100, and the difference is nitrogen-free-extract. In studying the nutritive value of foods, particular attention should be given to the nature of the nitrogen-free-extract, as in some instances it is composed of sugar and in others of starch, pectin, or pentosan (gum sugars). While all these compounds have practically the same fuel value, they differ in composition, structure, and the way in which they are acted upon by chemicals and digestive ferments.[1]

13. Fat.--Fat is found mainly in the seeds of plants, but to some extent in the leaves and stems. It differs from starch in containing more carbon and less oxygen. In starch there is about 44 per cent of carbon, while in fat there

is 75 per cent. Hence it is that when fat is burned or undergoes combustion, it yields a larger amount of the products of combustion--carbon dioxid and water--than does starch. A gram of fat produces 2-1/4 times as much heat as a gram of starch. Fat is the most concentrated non-nitrogenous nutrient. As found in food materials, it is a mechanical mixture of various fats, among which are stearin, palmitin, and olein. Stearin and palmitin are hard fats, crystalline in structure, and with a high melting point, while olein is a liquid. In addition to these three, there are also small amounts of other fats, as butyrin in butter, which give character or individuality to materials. There are a number of vegetable fats or oils which are used for food purposes and, when properly prepared and refined, have a high nutritive value. Occasionally one fat of cheaper origin but not necessarily of lower nutritive value is substituted for another. The fats have definite physical and chemical properties which enable them to be readily distinguished, as iodine number, specific gravity, index of refraction, and heat of combustion. By iodine number is meant the percentage of iodine that will unite chemically with the fat. Wheat oil has an iodine number of about 100, meaning that one pound of wheat oil will unite chemically with one pound of iodine. Fats have a lower specific gravity than water, usually ranging from .89 to .94, the specific gravity of a fat being fairly constant. All fats can be separated into glycerol and a fatty acid, glycerol or glycerine being common constituents, while each fat yields its own characteristic acid, as stearin, stearic acid; palmitin, palmitic acid; and olein, oleic acid. The fats are soluble in ether, chloroform, and benzine. In the chemical analysis of foods, they are separated with ether, and along with the fat, variable amounts of other substances are extracted, these extractive products usually being called "ether extract" or "crude fat."[5] The ether extract of plant tissue contains in addition to fat appreciable amounts of cellulose, gums, coloring, and other materials. From cereal products the ether extract is largely fat, but in some instances lecithin and other nitrogenous fatty substances are present, while in animal food products, as milk and meat, the ether extract is nearly pure fat.

14. Organic Acids.--Many vegetable foods contain small amounts of organic acids, as malic acid found in apples, citric in lemons, and tartaric in

grapes. These give characteristic taste to foods, but have no direct nutritive value. They do not yield heat and energy as do starch, fat, and protein; they are, however, useful for imparting flavor and palatability, and it is believed they promote to some extent the digestion of foods with which they are combined by encouraging the secretion of the digestive fluids. Many fruits and vegetables owe their dietetic value to the organic acids which they contain. In plants they are usually in chemical combination with the minerals, forming compounds as salts, or with the organic compounds, producing materials as acid proteins. In the plant economy they take an essential part in promoting growth and aiding the plant to secure by osmotic action its mineral food from the soil. Organic acids are found to some extent in animal foods, as the various lactic acids of meat and milk. They are also formed in food materials as the result of ferment action. When seeds germinate, small amounts of carbohydrates are converted into organic acids. In general the organic acids are not to be considered as nutrients, but as food adjuncts, increasing palatability and promoting digestion.

15. Essential Oils.--Essential or volatile oils differ from fats, or fixed oils, in chemical composition and physical properties.[6] The essential oils are readily volatilized, leaving no permanent residue, while the fixed fats are practically non-volatile. Various essential oils are present in small amounts in nearly all vegetable food materials, and the characteristic flavor of many fruits is due to them. It is these compounds which are used for flavoring purposes, as discussed in Chapter IV. The amount in a food material is very small, usually only a few hundredths of a per cent. The essential oils have no direct food value, but indirectly, like the organic acids, they assist in promoting favorable digestive action, and are also valuable because they impart a pleasant taste. Through poor methods of cooking and preparation, the essential oils are readily lost from some foods.

16. Mixed Compounds.--Food materials frequently contain compounds which do not naturally fall into the five groups mentioned,--carbohydrates, pectose substances, fats, organic acids, and essential oils. The amount of such compounds is small, and they are classed as miscellaneous or mixed

non-nitrogenous compounds. Some of them may impart a negative value to the food, and there are others which have all the characteristics, as far as general composition is concerned, of the non-nitrogenous compounds, but contain nitrogen, although as a secondary rather than an essential constituent.

17. Nutritive Value of Non-nitrogenous Compounds.--The non-nitrogenous compounds, taken as a class, are incapable alone of sustaining life, because they do not contain any nitrogen, and this is necessary for producing proteid material in the animal body. They are valuable for the production of heat and energy, and when associated with the nitrogenous compounds, are capable of forming non-nitrogenous reserve tissue. It is equally impossible to sustain life for any prolonged period with the nitrogenous compounds alone. It is when these two classes are properly blended and naturally united in food materials that their main value is secured. For nutrition purposes they are mutually related and dependent. Some food materials contain the nitrogenous and non-nitrogenous compounds blended in such proportion as to enable one food alone to practically sustain life, while in other cases it is necessary, in order to secure the best results in the feeding of animals and men, to combine different foods varying in their content of these two classes of compounds.[7]

NITROGENOUS COMPOUNDS

18. General Composition.--The nitrogenous compounds are more complex in composition than the non-nitrogenous. They are composed of a larger number of elements, united in different ways so as to form a much more complex molecular structure. Foods contain numerous nitrogenous organic compounds, which, for purposes of study, are divided into four divisions,-- proteids, albuminoids, amids, and alkaloids. In addition to these, there are other nitrogenous compounds which do not naturally fall into any one of the four divisions.

The material is digested in the flask (3) with sulphuric acid and the organic nitrogen converted into ammonium sulphate, which is later liberated and distilled at 1, and the ammonia neutralized with standard acid (2).]

Also in some foods there are small amounts of nitrogen in mineral forms, as nitrates and nitrites.

19. Protein.--The term "protein" is applied to a large class of nitrogenous compounds resembling each other in general composition, but differing widely in structural composition. As a class, the proteins contain about 16 per cent of nitrogen, 52 per cent of carbon, from 6 to 7 per cent of hydrogen, 22 per cent of oxygen, and less than 2 per cent of sulphur. These elements are combined in a great variety of ways, forming various groups or radicals. In studying the protein molecule a large number of derivative products have been observed, as amid radicals, various hydrocarbons, fatty acids, and carbohydrate-like bodies.[8] It would appear that in the chemical composition of the proteins there are all the constituents, or simpler products, of the non-nitrogenous compounds, and these are in chemical combination with amid radicals and nitrogen in various forms. The nitrogen of many proteids appears to be present in more than one form or radical. The proteids take an important part in life processes. They are found more extensively in animal than in plant bodies. The protoplasm of both the plant and animal cell is composed mainly of protein.

Proteids are divided into various subdivisions, as albumins, globulins, albuminates, proteoses and peptones, and insoluble proteids. In plant and animal foods a large amount of the protein is present as insoluble proteids; that is, they are not dissolved by solvents, as water and dilute salt solution. The albumins are soluble in water and coagulated by heat at a temperature of 157?to 161?F. Whenever a food material is soaked in water, the albumin is removed and can then be coagulated by the action of heat, or of chemicals, as tannic acid, lead acetate, and salts of mercury. The globulins are proteids extracted from food materials by dilute salt solution after the removal of the albumins. Globulins also are coagulated by heat and precipitated by chemicals. The amount of globulins in vegetable foods is small. In animal foods myosin in meat and vitellin, found in the yolk of the egg, and some of the proteids of the blood, are examples of globulins. Albuminates are casein-like proteids found in both animal and vegetable foods. They are supposed to be proteins that are in feeble chemical combination with acid and alkaline compounds, and they are sometimes called acid and alkali proteids. Some are precipitated from their solutions by acids and others by alkalies. Peas and beans contain quite large amounts of a casein-like proteid called legumin. Proteoses and peptones are proteins soluble in water, but not coagulated by heat. They are produced from other proteids by ferment action during the digestion of food and the germination of seeds, and are often due to the changes resulting from the action of the natural ferments or enzymes inherent in the food materials. As previously stated, the insoluble proteids are present in far the largest amount of any of the nitrogenous materials of foods. Lean meat and the gluten of wheat and other grains are examples of the insoluble proteids. The various insoluble proteids from different food materials each has its own composition and distinctive chemical and physical properties, and from each a different class and percentage amount of derivative products are obtained.[1] While in general it is held that the various proteins have practically the same nutritive value, it is possible that because differences in structural composition and the products formed during digestion there may exist notable differences in nutritive value. During digestion the insoluble proteids undergo an extended series of chemical changes. They are partially oxidized, and the nitrogenous portion of the molecule is eliminated mainly in the form of amids, as urea. The insoluble proteins constitute the main source of the nitrogenous food supply of both humans and animals.

20. Crude Protein.--In the analysis of foods, the term "crude protein" is used to designate the total nitrogenous compounds considered collectively; it is composed largely of protein, but also includes the amids, alkaloids, and albuminoids. "Crude protein" and "total nitrogenous compounds" are practically synonymous terms. The various proteins all contain about 16 per cent of nitrogen; that is, one part of nitrogen is equivalent to 6.25 parts of protein. In analyzing a food material, the total organic nitrogen is determined and the amount multiplied by 6.25 to obtain the crude protein. In some food

materials, as cereals, the crude protein is largely pure protein, while in others, as potatoes, it is less than half pure protein, the larger portion being amids and other compounds. In comparing the crude protein content of one food with that of another, the nature of both proteids should be considered and also the amounts of non-proteid constituents. The factor 6.25 for calculating the protein equivalent of foods is not strictly applicable to all foods. For example, the proteids of wheat--gliadin and glutenin--contain over 18 per cent of nitrogen, making the nitrogen factor about 5.68 instead of 6.25. If wheat contains 2 per cent of nitrogen, it is equivalent to 12.5 per cent of crude protein, using the factor 6.25; or to 11.4, using the factor 5.7. The nitrogen content of foods is absolute; the protein content is only relative.[9]

21. Food Value of Protein.--Because of its complexity in composition, protein is capable of being used by the body in a greater variety of ways than starch, sugar, or fat. In addition to producing heat and energy, protein serves the unique function of furnishing material for the construction of new muscular tissue and the repair of that which is worn out. It is distinctly a tissue-building nutrient. It also enters into the composition of all the vital fluids of the body, as the blood, chyme, chyle, and the various digestive fluids. Hence it is that protein is required as a nutrient by the animal body, and it cannot be produced from non-nitrogenous compounds. In vegetable bodies, the protein can be produced synthetically from amids, which in turn are formed from ammonium compounds. While protein is necessary in the ration, an excessive amount should be avoided. When there is more than is needed for functional purposes, it is used for heat and energy, and as foods rich in protein are usually the most expensive, an excess adds unnecessarily to the cost of the ration. Excess of protein in the ration may also result in a diseased condition, due to imperfect elimination of the protein residual products from the body.[10]

22. Albuminoids differ from proteids in general composition and, to some extent, in nutritive value. They are found in animal bodies mainly in the connective tissue and in the skin, hair, and nails. Some of the albuminoids, as nuclein, are equal in food value to protein, while others have a lower food

value. In general, albuminoids are capable of conserving the protein of the body, and hence are called "protein sparers," but they cannot in every way enter into the composition of the body, as do the true proteins.

23. Amids and Amines.--These are nitrogenous compounds of simpler structure than the proteins and albuminoids. They are sometimes called compound ammonia in that they are derived from ammonia by the replacement of one of the hydrogen atoms with an organic radical. In plants, amids are intermediate compounds in the production of the proteids, and in some vegetables a large portion of the nitrogen is amids. In animal bodies amids are formed during oxidation, digestion, and disintegration of proteids. It is not definitely known whether or not a protein in the animal body when broken down into amid form can again be reconstructed into protein. The amids have a lower food value than the proteids and albuminoids. It is generally held that, to a certain extent, they are capable, when combined with proteids, of preventing rapid conversion of the body proteid into soluble form. When they are used in large amounts in a ration, they tend to hasten oxidation rather than conservation of the proteids.

24. Alkaloids.--In some plant bodies there are small amounts of nitrogenous compounds called alkaloids. They are not found to any appreciable extent in food plants. The alkaloids, like ammonia, are basic in character and unite with acids to form salts. Many medicinal plants owe their value to the alkaloids which they contain. In animal bodies alkaloids are formed when the tissue undergoes fermentation changes, and also during disease, the products being known as ptomaines. Alkaloids have no food value, but act physiologically as irritants on the nerve centers, making them useful from a medicinal rather than from a nutritive point of view. To medical and pharmaceutical students the alkaloids form a very important group of compounds.

25. General Relationship of the Nitrogenous Compounds.--Among the various subdivisions of the nitrogenous compounds there exists a relationship similar to that among the non-nitrogenous compounds. From

proteids, amids and alkaloids may be formed, just as invert sugars and their products are formed from sucrose. Although glucose products are derived from sucrose, it is not possible to reverse the process and obtain sucrose or cane sugar from starch. So it is with proteins, while the amid may be obtained from the proteid in animal nutrition, as far as known the process cannot be reversed and proteids be obtained from amids. In the construction of the protein molecule of plants, nitrogen is absorbed from the soil in soluble forms, as compounds of nitrates and nitrites and ammonium salts. These are converted, first, into amids and then into proteids. In the animal body just the reverse of this process takes place,--the protein of the food undergoes a series of changes, and is finally eliminated from the body as an amid, which in turn undergoes oxidation and nitrification, and is converted into nitrites, nitrates, and ammonium salts. These forms of nitrogen are then ready to begin again in plant and animal bodies the same cycle of changes. Thus it is that nitrogen may enter a number of times into the composition of plant and animal tissues. Nature is very economical in her use of this element.[5]

CHAPTER II

CHANGES IN COMPOSITION OF FOODS DURING COOKING AND PREPARATION

26. Raw and Cooked Foods Compared.--Raw and cooked foods differ in chemical composition mainly in the content of water. The amount of nutrients on a dry matter basis is practically the same, but the structural composition is affected by cooking, and hence it is that a food prepared for the table often differs appreciably from the raw material. Cooked meat, for example, has not the same percentage and structural composition as raw meat, although the difference in nutritive value between a given weight of each is not large. During cooking, foods are acted upon chemically, physically, and bacteriologically, and it is usually the joint action of these three agencies that brings about the desirable changes incident to their preparation for the table.

27. Chemical Changes during Cooking.--Each of the chemical compounds of which foods are composed is influenced to a greater or less extent by heat and modified in composition. The chemistry of cooking is mainly a study of the chemical changes that take place when compounds, as cellulose, starch, sugar, pectin, fat, and the various proteids, are subjected to the joint action of heat, moisture, air, and ferments. The changes which affect the cellulose are physical rather than chemical. A slight hydration of the cellular tissue, however, does take place. In human foods cellulose is not found to any appreciable extent. Many vegetables, as potatoes, which are apparently composed of cellular substances, contain but little true cellulose. Starch, as previously stated, undergoes hydration in the presence of water, and, at a temperature of 120?C., is converted into dextrine. At a higher temperature disintegration of the starch molecule takes place, with the formation of carbon monoxid, carbon dioxid, and water, and the production of a residue richer in carbon than is starch. On account of the moisture, the temperature in many cooking operations is not sufficiently high for changes other than hydration and preliminary dextrinizing. In Chapter XI is given a more extended account of the changes affecting starch which occur in bread making.

During the cooking process sugars undergo inversion to a slight extent. That is, sucrose is converted into levulose and dextrose sugars. At a higher temperature, sugar is broken up into its constituents--water and carbon dioxide. The organic acids which many fruits and vegetables contain hasten the process of inversion. When sugar is subjected to dry heat, it becomes a brown, caramel-like material sometimes called barley sugar. During cooking, sugars are not altered in solubility or digestibility; starches, however, are changed to a more soluble form, and pectin--a jelly-like substance--is converted from a less to a more soluble condition, as stated in Chapter I. Changes incident to the cooking of fruits and vegetables rich in pectin, as in the making of jellies, are similar to those which take place in the last stages of ripening.

The fats are acted upon to a considerable extent by heat. Some of the vegetable oils undergo slight oxidation, resulting in decreased solubility in ether, but since there is no volatilization of the fatty matter, it is a change that does not materially affect the total fuel value of the food.[11]

There is a general tendency for the proteids to become less soluble by the action of heat, particularly the albumins and globulins. The protein molecule dissociates at a high temperature, with formation of volatile products, and therefore foods rich in protein should not be subjected to extreme heat, as losses of food value may result. During cooking, proteids undergo hydration, which is necessary and preliminary to digestion, and the heating need be carried only to this point, and not to the splitting up of the molecule. Prolonged high temperature in the cooking of proteids and starches is unnecessary in order to induce the desired chemical changes. When these nutrients are hydrated, they are in a condition to undergo digestion, without the body being compelled to expend unnecessary energy in bringing about this preliminary change. Hence it is that, while proper cooking does not materially affect the total digestibility of proteids or starches, it influences ease of digestion, as well as conserves available energy, thereby making more economical use of these nutrients.

28. Physical Changes.--The mechanical structure of foods is influenced by cooking to a greater extent than is the chemical composition. One of the chief objects of cooking is to bring the food into better mechanical condition for digestion.[12] Heat and water cause partial disintegration of both animal and vegetable tissues. The cell-cementing materials are weakened, and a softening of the tissues results. Often the action extends still further in vegetable foods, resulting in disintegration of the individual starch granules. When foods are subjected to dry heat, the moisture they contain is converted into steam, which causes bursting of the tissues. A good example of this is the popping of corn. Heat may result, too, in mechanical removal of some of the nutrients, as the fats, which are liquefied at temperatures ranging from 100?to 200?F. Many foods which in the raw state contain quite large amounts of fat, lose a portion mechanically during cooking, as is the case

with bacon when it is cut in thin slices and fried or baked until crisp. When foods are boiled, the natural juices being of somewhat different density from the water in which they are cooked, slight osmotic changes occur. There is a tendency toward equalization of the composition of the juices of the food and the water in which they are cooked. In order to achieve the best mechanical effects in cooking, high temperatures are not necessary, except at first for rupturing the tissues; softening of the tissues is best effected by prolonged and slow heat. At a higher temperature many of the volatile and essential oils are lost, while at lower temperatures these are retained and in some instances slightly developed. The cooking should be sufficiently prolonged and the temperature high enough to effectually disintegrate and soften all of the tissues, but not to cause extended chemical changes.

There is often an unnecessarily large amount of heat lost through faulty construction of stoves and lack of judicious use of fuels, which greatly enhances the cost of preparing foods. Ovens are frequently coated with deposits of soot; this causes the heat to be thrown out into the room or lost through the chimney, rather than utilized for heating the oven. In an ordinary cook stove it is estimated that less than 7 per cent of the heat and energy of the fuel is actually employed in bringing about physical and chemical changes incident to cooking.[13]

29. Bacteriological Changes.--The bacterial organisms of foods are destroyed in the cooking, provided a temperature of 150?F. is reached and maintained for several minutes. The interior of foods rarely reaches a temperature above 200?F., because of the water they contain which is not completely removed below 212? One of the chief objects in cooking food is to render it sterile. Not only do bacteria become innocuous through cooking, but various parasites, as trichina and tapeworm, are destroyed, although some organisms can live at a comparatively high temperature. Cooked foods are easily re-inoculated, in some cases more readily than fresh foods, because they are in a more disintegrated condition.

In many instances bacteria are of material assistance in the preparation of foods, as in bread making, butter making, curing of cheese, and ripening of meat. All the chemical compounds of which foods are composed are subject to fermentation, each compound being acted upon by its special ferment body. Those which convert the proteids into soluble form, as the peptonizing ferments, have no action upon the carbohydrates. A cycle of bacteriological changes often takes place in a food material, one class of ferments working until their products accumulate to such an extent as to prevent their further activity, and then the process is taken up by others, as they find the conditions favorable for development. This change of bacterial flora in food materials is akin to the changes in the vegetation occupying soils. In each case, there is a constant struggle for possession. Bacteria take a much more important part in the preparation of foods than is generally considered. As a result of their workings, various chemical products, as organic acids and aromatic compounds, are produced. The organic acids chemically unite with the nutrients of foods, changing their composition and physical properties. Man is, to a great extent, dependent upon bacterial action. Plant life also is dependent upon the bacterial changes which take place in the soil and in the plant tissues. The stirring of seeds into activity is apparently due to enzymes or soluble ferments which are inherent in the seed. A study of the bacteriological changes which foods undergo in their preparation and digestion more properly belongs to the subject of bacteriology, and in this work only brief mention is made of some of the more important parts which microoganisms take in the preparation of foods.

30. Insoluble Ferments.--Insoluble ferments are minute, plant-like bodies of definite form and structure, and can be studied only with the microscope.[1] They are developed from spores or seeds, or from the splitting or budding of the parent cells. Under suitable conditions they multiply rapidly, deriving the energy for their life processes from the chemical changes which they induce. For example, in the souring of milk the milk sugar is changed by the lactic acid ferments into lactic acid. In causing chemical changes, the ferment gives none of its own material to the reacting substance. These ferment bodies undergo life processes similar to plants of a higher order.

All foods contain bacteria or ferments. In fact, it is impossible for a food stored and prepared under ordinary conditions, unless it has been specially treated, to be free from them. Some of them are useful, some are injurious, while others are capable of producing disease. The objectionable bacteria are usually destroyed by the joint action of sunlight, pure air, and water.

31. Soluble Ferments.--Many plant and animal cells have the power of secreting substances soluble in water and capable of producing fermentation changes; to these the term "soluble ferments," or "enzymes," is applied. These ferments have not a cell structure like the organized ferments. When germinated seed, as malted barley, is extracted, a soluble and highly nitrogenous substance, called the diastase ferment, is secured that changes starch into soluble forms. The soluble ferments induce chemical change by causing molecular disturbance or splitting up of the organic compounds, resulting in the production of derivative products. They take an important part in animal and plant nutrition, as by their action insoluble compounds are brought into a soluble condition so they can be utilized for nutritive purposes. In many instances ferment changes are due to the joint action of soluble and insoluble ferments. The insoluble ferment secretes an enzyme which induces a chemical change, modified by the further action of the soluble ferment. Many of the enzymes carry on their work at a low temperature, as in the curing of meat and cheese in cold storage.[14]

32. General Relationship of Chemical, Physical, and Bacteriological Changes.--It cannot be said that the beneficial results derived from the cooking of foods are due to either chemical, physical, or bacteriological change alone, but to the joint action of the three. In order to secure a chemical change, a physical change must often precede, and a bacteriological change cannot take place without causing a change in chemical composition; the three are closely related and interdependent.

33. Esthetic Value of Foods.--Foods should be not only of good physical texture and contain the requisite nutrients, but they should also be pleasing to the eye and served in the most attractive manner. Some foods owe a part

of their commercial value to color, and when they are lacking in natural color they are not consumed with a relish. There is no objection to the addition of coloring matter to foods, provided it is of a non-injurious character and does not affect the amount of nutrients, and that its presence and the kind of coloring material are made known. Some foods contain objectionable colors which are eliminated during the process of manufacture, as in the case of sugar and flour. As far as removal of coloring matter from foods during refining is concerned, there can be no objection, so long as no injurious reagents or chemicals are retained, as the removal of the color in no way affects the nutritive value or permits fraud, but necessitates higher purification and refining. The use of chemicals and reagents in the preparation and refining of foods is considered permissible in all cases where the reagents are removed by subsequent processes. In the food decisions of the United States Department of Agriculture, it is stated: "Not excluded under this provision are substances properly used in the preparation of food products for clarification or refining and eliminated in the further process of manufacture." [15]

CHAPTER III

VEGETABLE FOODS

34. General Composition.--Vegetable foods, with the exception of cereals, legumes, and nuts, contain a smaller percentage of protein than animal food products. They vary widely in composition and nutritive value; in some, starch predominates, while in others, sugar, cellulose, and pectin bodies are most abundant. The general term "vegetable foods" is used in this work to include roots, tubers, garden vegetables, cereals, legumes, and all prepared foods of vegetable origin.

35. Potatoes contain about 75 per cent of water and 25 per cent of dry matter, the larger portion being starch. There is but little nitrogenous material in the potato, only 2.25 per cent, of which about half is in the form of proteids. There are ten parts of non-nitrogenous substance to every one

part of nitrogenous; or, in other words, the potato has a wide nutritive ratio, and as an article of diet needs to be supplemented with foods rich in protein. The mineral matter, cellular tissue, and fat in potatoes are small in amount, as are also the organic acids. Mechanically considered, the potato is composed of three parts,--outer skin, inner skin, and flesh. The layer immediately beneath the outer skin is slightly colored, and is designated the fibro-vascular layer. The outer and inner skins combined make up about 10 per cent of the weight of the potato.

A large portion of the protein of the potato is albumin, which is soluble in water. When potatoes are peeled, cut in small pieces, and soaked in water for several hours before boiling, 80 per cent of the crude protein, or total nitrogenous material, is extracted, rendering the product less valuable as food. When potatoes are placed directly in boiling water, the losses of nitrogenous compounds are reduced to about 7 per cent, and, when the skins are not removed, to 1 per cent. Digestion experiments show that 92 per cent of the starch and 72 per cent of the protein are digested.[12] Compared with other foods, potatoes are often a cheap source of non-nitrogenous nutrients. If used in excessive amounts, however, they have a tendency to make the ration unbalanced and too bulky.

MECHANICAL COMPOSITION OF THE POTATO

== |Per Cent Unpeeled potatoes | 100.0 Outer, or true skin | 2.5 Inner skin, or fibro-vascular layer[A] | 8.5 Flesh | 89.0

==

CHEMICAL COMPOSITION OF THE POTATO

==

========== | | | | CARBOHYDRATES |-----|-------|---|------------------------ |Water| Crude |Fat|Nitrogen-free-| | | |Protein| | extract |Fiber|Ash | % | % | % | %

| % |% --------------------|-----|-------|---|--------------|-----|--- Outer, or true skin | 80.1| 2.7 |0.8| 14.|6 |1.8 Inner skin, or |||||| fibro-vascular |||||| layer | 83.2| 2.3 |0.1| 12.6 | 0.7 |1.1 Flesh | 81.1| 2.0 |0.1| 15.7 | 0.3 |0.8 Average of 86 |||||| American analyses[B]| 78.0| 2.2 |0.1| 18.|8 |0.9 Average of 118 |||| | | European analyses[C]| 75.0| 2.1 |0.1| 21.0 | 0.7 |1.1

==

===========

[Footnote A: Including a small amount of flesh.]

[Footnote B: From an unpublished compilation of analyses of American food products.]

36. Sweet Potatoes contain more dry matter than white potatoes, the difference being due mainly to the presence of about 6 per cent of sugar. There is approximately the same starch content, but more fat, protein, and fiber. As a food, they supply a large amount of non-nitrogenous nutrients.

37. Carrots contain about half as much dry matter as potatoes, and half of the dry matter is sugar, nearly equally divided between sucrose and levulose, or fruit sugar. Like the potato, carrots have some organic acids and a relatively small amount of proteids. In carrots and milk there is practically the same per cent of water. The nutrients in each, however, differ both as to kind and proportion. Experiments with the cooking of carrots show that if a large amount of water is used, 30 per cent or more of the nutrients, particularly of the more soluble sugar and albumin, are extracted and lost in the drain waters.[12] The color of the carrot is due to the non-nitrogenous compound carrotin, $C_{26}H_{38}$. Carrots are valuable in a ration not because of the nutrients they supply, but for the palatability and the mechanical action which the vegetable fiber exerts upon the process of digestion.

38. Parsnips contain more solid matter than beets or carrots, of which 3 to 4 per cent is starch. The starch grains are very small, being only about one

twentieth the size of the potato starch grains. There is 3 per cent of sugar and an appreciable amount of fat, more than in any other of the vegetables of this class, and seven times as much as in the potato. The mineral matter is of somewhat different nature from that in potatoes; in parsnips one half is potash and one quarter phosphoric acid, while in potatoes three quarters are potash and one fifth phosphoric acid.

39. Cabbage contains very little dry matter, usually less than 10 per cent. It is proportionally richer in nitrogenous compounds than many vegetables, as about two of the ten parts of dry matter are crude protein, which makes the nutritive ratio one to five. During cooking 30 to 40 per cent of the nutrients are extracted. Cabbage imparts to the ration bulk but comparatively little nutritive material. It is a valuable food adjunct, particularly used raw, as in a salad, when it is easily digested and retains all of the nutrients.[12]

40. Cauliflower has much the same general composition as cabbage, from which it differs mainly in mechanical structure.

41. Beets.--The garden beet contains a little more protein than carrots, but otherwise has about the same general composition, and the statements made in regard to the losses of nutrients in the cooking of carrots and to their use in the dietary apply also to beets.

42. Cucumbers contain about 4 per cent of dry matter. The amount of nutrients is so small as to scarcely allow them to be considered a food. They are, however, a valuable food adjunct, as they impart palatability.

43. Lettuce contains about 7 per cent of solids, of which 1.5 is protein and 2.5 starch and sugar. While low in nutrients, it is high in dietetic value, because of the chlorophyll which it contains. It has been suggested that it is valuable, too, for supplying iron in an organic form, as there is iron chemically combined with the chlorophyll.

44. Onions are aromatic bulbs, valuable for condimental rather than

nutritive purposes. They contain essential and volatile oils, which impart characteristic odor and flavor. In the onion there are about 1.5 per cent of protein and 9.5 per cent of non-nitrogenous material. Onions are often useful in stimulating the digestive tract to action.

45. Spinach is a valuable food, not to be classed merely as a relish. Its composition is interesting; for, although there is 90 per cent water, and less than 10 per cent dry matter, it still possesses high food value. Spinach contains 2.1 per cent crude protein, or about one part to every four parts of carbohydrates. In potatoes, turnips, and beets there are ten or more parts of carbohydrates to every one part of protein.

46. Asparagus is composed largely of water, about 93 per cent. The dry matter, however, is richer in protein than that of many vegetables. Asparagus contains, too, an amid compound, asparagin, which gives some of the characteristics to the vegetable.

47. Melons.--Melons contain from 8 to 10 per cent of dry matter, the larger portion of which is sugar and allied carbohydrates. The flavor is due to small amounts of essential oils and to organic acids associated with the sugars. Melons possess condimental rather than nutritive value.

48. Tomatoes.--The tomato belongs to the night-shade family, and for this reason was long looked upon with suspicion. It was first used for ornamental purposes and was called "love-apple." Gradually, as the idea of its poisonous nature became dispelled, it grew more and more popular as a food, until now in the United States it is one of the most common garden vegetables. It contains 7 per cent of dry matter, 4 per cent of which is sucrose, dextrose, and levulose. It also contains some malic acid, and a small amount of proteids, amids, cellulose, and coloring material. In the canning of tomatoes, if too much of the juice is excluded, a large part of the nutritive material is lost, as the sugars and albumins are all soluble and readily removed.[16] If the seeds are objectionable, they may be removed by straining and the juice added to the fleshy portion. The product then has a higher nutritive value

than if the juice had been discarded with the seeds.

49. Sweet Corn.--Fresh, soft, green, sweet corn contains about 75 per cent of water. The dry matter is half starch and one quarter sugar. The protein content makes up nearly 5 per cent, a larger proportional amount than is found in the ripened corn, due to the fact that the proteids are deposited in the early stages of growth and the carbohydrates mainly in the last stages. Sweet corn is a vegetable of high nutritive value and palatability.

50. Eggplant contains a high per cent of water,--90 per cent. The principal nutrients are starch and sugar, which make up about half the weight of the dry matter. It does not itself supply a large amount of nutrients, but the way in which it is prepared, by combination with butter, bread crumbs, and eggs, makes it a nutritious and palatable dish, the food value being derived mainly from the materials with which it is combined, the eggplant giving the flavor and palatability.

51. Squash and Pumpkin.--Squash has much the same general composition and food value as beets and carrots, although it belongs to a different family. Pumpkins contain less dry matter than squash. The dry matter of both is composed largely of starch and sugar and, like many other of the vegetables, they are often combined with food materials containing a large amount of nutrients, as in pumpkin and squash pies, where the food value is derived mainly from the milk, sugar, eggs, flour, and butter or other shortening used.

52. Celery.--The dry matter of celery is comparatively rich in nitrogenous material, although the amount is small, and the larger proportion is in non-proteid form. When grown on rich soil, celery may contain an appreciable quantity of nitrates and nitrites, which have not been converted into amids and proteids. The supposed medicinal value is probably due to the nitrites which are generally present. Celery is valuable from a dietetic rather than a nutritive point of view.

53. Sanitary Condition of Vegetables.--The conditions under which

vegetables are grown have much to do with their value, particularly from a sanitary point of view. Uncooked vegetables often cause the spread of diseases, particularly those, as cholera and typhoid, affecting the digestive tract. Particles of dirt containing the disease-producing organisms adhere to the uncooked vegetable and find their way into the digestive tract, where the bacteria undergo incubation. When sewage has been used for fertilizing the land, as in sewage irrigation, the vegetables are unsound from a sanitary point of view. Such vegetables should be thoroughly cleaned and also well cooked, in order to render them sterile. Vegetables to be eaten in the raw state should be dipped momentarily into boiling water, to destroy the activity of the germs present upon the surface. They may then be immediately immersed in ice-cold water, to preserve the crispness.

54. Miscellaneous Compounds in Vegetables.--In addition to the general nutrients which have been discussed, many of the vegetables contain some tannin, glucosides, and essential oils; and occasionally those grown upon rich soils have appreciable amounts of nitrogen compounds, as nitrates and nitrites, which have not been built up into proteids. Vegetables have a unique value in the dietary, and while as a class they contain small amounts of nutrients, they are indispensable for promoting health and securing normal digestion of the food.

55. Canned Vegetables.--When sound vegetables are thoroughly cooked to destroy ferments, and then sealed in cans while hot, they can be kept for a long time without any material impairment of nutritive value. During the cooking process there is lost a part of the essential oils, which gives a slightly different flavor to the canned or tinned goods.[17] In some canned vegetables preservatives are used, but the enactment and enforcement of national and state laws have greatly reduced their use. When the cans are made of a poor quality of tin, or the vegetables are of high acidity, some of the metal is dissolved in sufficient quantity to be objectionable from a sanitary point of view.[18]

56. Edible Portion and Refuse of Vegetables.--Many vegetables have

appreciable amounts of refuse,[19] or non-edible parts, as skin, pods, seeds, and pulp, and in determining the nutritive value, these must be considered, as in some cases less than 50 per cent of the weight of the material is edible portion, which proportionally increases the cost of the nutrients. Ordinarily, the edible part is richer in protein than the entire material as purchased. In some cases, however, the refuse is richer in protein, but the protein is in a less available form. See comparison of potatoes and potato skins.

CHAPTER IV

FRUITS, FLAVORS, AND EXTRACTS

57. General Composition.--Fruits are characterized by containing a large amount of water and only a small amount of dry matter, which is composed mainly of sugar and non-nitrogenous compounds. Fruits contain but little fatty material and protein. A large portion of the total nitrogen is in the form of amid compounds. Organic acids, as citric, tartaric, and malic, are found in all fruits, and the essential oils form a characteristic feature. The taste of fruits is due mainly to the blending of the various organic acids, essential oils, and sugars. Although fruits contain a high per cent of water, they are nevertheless valuable as food.[20] The constituents present to the greatest extent are sugars and acids. The sugar is not all like the common granulated sugar, but in ripe fruits a part is in the form known as levulose or fruit sugar, which is two and a half times sweeter than granulated sugar. Sugars are valuable for heat-and fat-producing purposes, but not for muscle repairing. Proteids are the muscle-forming nutrients. The organic acids, as malic acid in apples, citric acid in lemons and oranges, and tartaric acid in grapes, have characteristic medicinal properties. The sugar, proteid, and acid content of some of our more common fruits is given in the following table:[21]

COMPOSITION OF FRUITS

	WATER	PROTEIDS	SUGAR	ACID IN JUICE	KIND OF ACID
	Per Cent	Per Cent	Per Cent	Per Cent	
Apples (Baldwin)	85.0	0.50	10.75	0.92	Malic
Apples, sweet	86.0	0.50	11.75	0.20	Malic
Blackberries	88.9	0.90	11.50	0.75	Malic
Currants	86.0	--	1.96	5.80	Tartaric
Grapes	83.0	1.50	10 to 16	1.2 to 5	Tartaric
Strawberries	90.8	0.95	5.36	1.40	Malic
Oranges	85.0	1.10	10.00	1.30	Citric
Lemons	84.0	0.95	2.00	7.20	Citric

In addition to sugars, acids, and proteids, there are a great many other compounds in fruits. Those which give the characteristic taste are called essential or volatile oils.

58. Food Value.--When the nutrients alone are considered, fruits appear to have a low food value, but they should not be judged entirely on this basis, because they impart palatability and flavor to other foods and exercise a favorable influence upon the digestive process. In the human ration fruits are a necessary adjunct.

59. Apples.--Apples vary in composition with the variety and physical characteristics of the fruit. In general they contain from 10 to 16 per cent of dry matter, of which 75 per cent, or more, is sugar or allied carbohydrates. Among the organic acids malic predominates, and the acidity ranges from 0.1 to 0.8 per cent. Apples contain but little protein, less than 1 per cent. There is some pectin, or jelly-like substance closely related to the carbohydrates. The flavor of the apple varies with the content of sugar, organic acids, and essential oils. During storage some apples appear to undergo further ripening, resulting in partial inversion of the sucrose, and there is a slight loss of weight, due to the formation of carbon dioxide. The apple is an important and valuable adjunct to the dietary.[22]

60. Oranges contain nearly the same proportion of dry matter as apples, the

larger part of which is sugar. Citric acid predominates and ranges in different varieties from 1 to 2.5 per cent. The amounts of protein, fat, and cellulose are small. In some varieties of oranges there is more iron and sulphur than is usually found in fruits. All fruits, however, contain small amounts, but not as much as is found in green vegetables. The average composition of oranges is as follows:

===
===== PHYSICAL COMPOSITION|CHEMICAL COMPOSITION OF EDIBLE PORTION --- Per Cent| Per Cent Rind 20 to 30| Solids 10 to 16 Pulp 25 to 35| Sugars 8 to 12 Juice 35 to 50| Citric acid 1 to 2.5 | Ash 0.5
===
=====

61. Lemons differ from oranges in containing more citric acid and less sucrose, levulose, and dextrose. The ash of the lemon is somewhat similar in general composition to the ash of the orange, but is larger in amount. The average composition of the lemon is as follows:

===
===== PHYSICAL COMPOSITION|CHEMICAL COMPOSITION OF EDIBLE PORTION --- Per Cent| Per Cent Rind 25 to 35| Solids 10 to 12 Pulp 25 to 35| Sugar 2 to 4 Juice 40 to 55| Citric acid 6 to 9
===
=====

62. Grape Fruit.--The rind and seed of this fruit make up about 25 per cent, leaving 75 per cent as edible portion. The juice contains 14 per cent solids, of which nearly 10 per cent is sugar and 2.5 per cent is citric acid. There is more acid in grape fruit than in oranges and appreciably less than in lemons.

The characteristic flavor is due to a glucoside-like material. Otherwise the composition and food value are about the same as of oranges.

63. Strawberries contain from 8 to 12 per cent of dry matter, mainly sugar and malic acid. The protein, fat, and ash usually make up less than 2 per cent. Essential oils and coloring substances are present in small amounts. It has been estimated that it would require 75 pounds of strawberries to supply the protein for a daily ration. Nevertheless they are valuable in the dietary. It has been suggested that the malic and other acids have antiseptic properties which, added to the appearance and palatability, make them a desirable food adjunct. Strawberries have high dietetic rather than high food value.

64. Grapes contain more dry matter than apples or oranges. There is no appreciable amount of protein or fat, and while they add some nutrients, as sugar, to the ration, they do not contribute any quantity. Their value, as in the case of other fruits, is due to palatability and indirect effect upon the digestibility of other foods. In the juice of grapes there is from 10 to 15 per cent or more of sugar, as sucrose, levulose, and dextrose. Grapes contain also from 1 to 1.5 per cent of tartaric acid, which, during the process of manufacture into wine, is rendered insoluble by the alcohol formed, and the product, known as argole, is used in the preparation of cream of tartar. Differences in flavor and taste of grapes are due to variations in the sugar, acid, and essential oil content.

65. Peaches contain about 12 per cent of dry matter, of which over 10 per cent is sugar and other carbohydrates. There is less than 1.5 per cent of protein, fat, and mineral matter and about 0.5 per cent of acid. The peach contains also a very small amount of hydrocyanic acid, which is more liberally present in the kernel than in the fruit. Flavor is imparted mainly by the sugar and essential oils. Peaches vary in composition with variety and environment.[23]

66. Plums contain the most dry matter of any of the fruits, about 22 per cent, mainly sugar. About one per cent is acid and about 0.5 per cent are protein

and ash. There are a great many varieties of plums, varying in composition. Dried plums (prunes) have mildly laxative properties.

67. Olives.--The ripe olive contains about 15 per cent of oil, exclusive of the pit, which makes up 20 per cent of the weight. In green, preserved olives there is considerably less oil. Because of the oil the olive has food value. Olive oil is slightly laxative and assists mechanically in the digestion of foods.

68. Figs.--Dried figs contain about 50 per cent of sugar and 3.5 per cent of protein. The fig has a mildly laxative action.

69. Dried Fruits.--Many fruits are prepared for market by drying. The dried fruit has a slightly different composition from the fresh fruit because of loss of the volatile and essential oils, and minor chemical changes which take place during the drying process. When free from preservatives, dried fruits are valuable adjuncts to the dietary and can be advantageously used when fresh fruits are not obtainable.

70. Canning and Preservation of Fruits.--To obtain the best results in canning, the fruit should not be overripe. After the ripened state has been reached fermentation and bacterial changes occur, and it is more difficult to preserve the fruit than when not so fully matured.[24] When a fruit has begun to ferment, it is hard to destroy the ferment bodies and their spores so as to prevent further ferment action. The chemical changes that occur in the last stages of ripening are similar to those which take place during the cooking process whereby the pectin or jelly-like substances are rendered more soluble and digestible.

71. Adulterated Canned Fruits.--Analyses of a number of canned fruits, made by various Boards of Health, show the presence of small amounts of arsenic, tin, lead, and other poisonous metals. The quantity dissolved depends upon the kind, age, and condition of the canned goods and the state of the fruit when canned. The longer a can of fruit or vegetable has been

kept in stock, the larger is the amount of tin or metal that has been dissolved. When fresh canned, there is usually very little dissolved tin, but in old goods the amount may be comparatively large. The tin used for the can is occasionally of poor quality and may contain some arsenic, which also is dissolved. The occasional use of canned goods preserved in tin is not objectionable, but they should not be used continually if it can be avoided. Preservatives, as borax, salicylic acid, benzoic acid, and sodium sulphate, are sometimes added to prevent fermentation and to preserve the natural appearance of the fruit or vegetable.[18]

72. Fruit Flavors and Extracts.--Formerly all fruit extracts and flavors were obtained from vegetable sources; at present many are made in the chemical laboratory by synthetic methods; that is, by combining simpler organic compounds and radicals to produce the material having the desired flavor and odor. The various fruit flavors are definite chemical compounds, and can be produced in the laboratory as well as in the cells of plants. When properly made, there is no difference in chemical composition between the two. As prepared in the laboratory, however, traces of acids, alkalies, and other compounds, used in bringing about the necessary chemical combination, are often present, not having been perfectly removed. Hence it is that natural and artificial flavors differ mainly in the impurities which the artificial flavors may contain.

Some of the flavoring materials have characteristic medicinal properties, as the flavor of bitter almond, which contains hydrocyanic acid, a poisonous substance. Flavors and extracts should not be indiscriminately used. In small amounts they often exert a favorable influence upon the digestion of foods, and the value of some fruits is in a large measure due to the special flavors they contain. A study of the separate compounds which impart flavor to fruits, as the various aldehydes, ethers, and organic salts, belongs to organic chemistry rather than to foods. Some of the simpler compounds of which flavors are composed may exist in entirely different form or combination in food products; as for example, pineapple flavoring is ethyl butrate. This can be prepared by combination of butyric acid from stale butter with alcohol which supplies the ethyl radical. The chemical union of the two produces the new compound, ethyl butrate, the distinctive flavoring substance of the pineapple. Banana flavor can be made from stale butter, caustic soda, and chloroform. None of these materials, as such, go into the flavor, but an essential radical is taken from each. These manufactured products, when properly made, are in every essential similar to the flavor made by the plant and stored up in the fruit. The plant combines the material in the laboratory of the plant cell, and the manufacturer of essences puts together these same constituents in a chemical laboratory. In the fruit, however, the essential oil is associated with a number of other compounds.

CHAPTER V

SUGARS, MOLASSES, SYRUP, HONEY, AND CONFECTIONS

73. Composition of Sugars.--The term "sugar" is applied to a large class of compounds composed of the elements carbon, hydrogen, and oxygen. Sugars used for household purposes are derived mainly from the sugar cane and the sugar beet.[25] At the present time about two fifths are obtained from the cane and about three fifths from the beet. When subjected to the same degree of refining, there is no difference in the chemical composition of the sugars from the two sources; they are alike in every respect and the chemist is unable to determine their origin. The production of sugar is an agricultural industry; the methods of manufacture pertain more to industrial chemistry than to the chemistry of foods, and therefore a discussion of them is omitted in this work.[26]

74. Commercial Grades of Sugar.--Sugars are graded according to the size of the granule, the color and general appearance of the crystals, and the per cent of sucrose or pure sugar. Common granulated sugar is from 98.5 to 99.7 per cent pure sucrose. The impurities consist mainly of moisture and mineral matter. In the process of refining, sulphur fumes are frequently used for bleaching and clarifying the solution.[26] The sulphurous acid formed is neutralized with lime, which is rendered insoluble and practically all

removed in subsequent filtrations. There are, however, traces of sulphates and sulphites in ordinary sugar, but these are in such small amounts as not to be injurious to health. When sugar is burned, as in the bomb calorimeter, so as to permit collection of all of the products of combustion, granulated sugar yields about 0.01 of a per cent of sulphur dioxid.[13] Occasionally coloring substances, as a small amount of indigo, are added to yellow tinged sugars to impart a white color, much on the same principle as the bluing of clothes. The amount used is usually extremely small, and the effect on health has never been determined. Occasionally, however, bluing is used to such an extent that a blue scum appears when the sugar is boiled with water. Sugar has high value for the production of heat and energy. Digestion experiments show that when it is used in the dietary in not excessive amounts, it is directly absorbed by the body and practically all available. It can advantageously be combined with other foods to form a part of the ration.[27] When a ration contains the requisite amount of protein, sugar is used to the best advantage. Alone it is incapable of sustaining life, because it does not contain any nitrogen. When sugar was substituted for an excess of protein in a ration, it was found to produce heat and energy at much less expense. Many foods, as apples, grapes, and small fruits, contain appreciable amounts of sugar and owe their food value almost entirely to their sugar content. In the dietary, sugar is too frequently regarded as a condiment instead of a nutrient, to be used for imparting palatability rather than for purposes of nutrition. While valuable for improving the taste of foods, the main worth of sugar is as a nutritive substance; used in the preparation of foods it adds to the total heat and energy of the ration. Sugar is sometimes used in excessive amounts and, as is the case with any food or nutrient, when that occurs, nutrition disturbances result, due to misuse of the food. Statistics show that the average consumption of sugar in the United States is nearly 70 pounds a year per capita. In the dietary of the adult, sugar to the extent of four ounces per day can be consumed advantageously. The exclusion of sugar from the diet of children is a great mistake, as they need it for heat and energy and to conserve the protein for growth.

"Sugar is one of the most important forms in which carbohydrates can be added to the diet of children. The great reduction in the price of sugar which has taken place in recent years is probably one of the causes of the improved physique of the rising generation. The fear that sugar may injure children's teeth is, largely illusory. The negroes who live largely on sugar cane have the finest teeth the world can show. If injudiciously taken, sugar may, however, injure the child's appetite and digestion. The craving for sweets which children show is no doubt the natural expression of a physiological need, but they should be taken with, and not between, meals."[28]

75. Sugar in the Dietary.--Sugar has an important place in the dietary. It not only serves for the production of heat and energy in the body, but is also valuable in enabling the proteids to be used more economically. In reasonable amounts, it is particularly valuable in the dietary of growing children, as the proteids of the food are then utilized to better advantage for growth. The unique value of sugar depends upon its intelligent use and its proper combination with other foods, particularly with those rich in the nitrogenous compounds or proteids. Sugar alone is incapable of sustaining life, but combined with other foods is a valuable nutrient. The amount which can be advantageously used depends largely upon the individual. Ordinarily three to five ounces per day is sufficient, although some persons cannot safely consume as much as this. In the case of diabetes mellitus, the amount of sugar in the ration must be materially reduced. Persons in normal health and engaged in outdoor work can use sugar to advantage.[29] Many of the "harvest drinks," made largely from molasses with a little ginger, and used extensively in some localities, are not without merit, as they contain an appreciable amount of nutrients. Milk contains more sugar as lactose or milk sugar than any other nutrient.

The craving for sugar by growing children and athletes is natural. Sugar, however, is often injudiciously used, and a perverted taste may be established which can be satisfied only by excessive amounts. This results in impaired digestion and malnutrition.

76. Maple Sugar.--Sugar obtained by evaporation from the sap of the maple

tree (Acer saccharinum) is identical, except for the foreign substances which it contains, with that from the beet and sugar cane. The mottled appearance and characteristic color and taste of maple sugar are due to the various organic acids and other compounds present in the maple sap and recovered in the sugar. Maple sugar, as ordinarily prepared, has 0.4 of a per cent or more of ash or mineral matter, while refined cane sugar contains less than one tenth as much.[30] Hence, when maple sugar is adulterated with cane and beet sugars, the ash content is noticeably lowered, as is also the content of organic acids. It is difficult, however, to determine with absolute certainty pure high grade maple sugar from the impure low grade to which a small amount of granulated sugar has been added.

77. Adulteration of Sugar.--Sugar at the present time is not materially adulterated. Other than the substances mentioned which are used for clarification and color, none are added during refining which remain in the sugar in appreciable amounts. Sugar does not readily lend itself to adulteration, as it has a definite crystalline structure, and materials that would be suitable for its adulteration are of entirely different physical character.[31] Cane sugar is not easily blended with glucose, or starch sugar, because of the physical differences between the two. The question of the kind of sugar to use in the household, as granulated, loaf, or pulverized, is largely one of personal choice, as there is no appreciable difference in the nutritive value or purity of the different kinds.

78. Dextrose Sugars.--Products known as glucose and dextrose sugars are made from corn and other starches; they can also be prepared from cane sugar by the use of heat, chemicals, or ferments for carrying on the process known as inversion. The dextrose sugars differ from cane sugar in containing a dissimilar number of carbon, hydrogen, and oxygen atoms in the molecule. The formula of the dextrose sugars is $C_6H_{12}O_6$, while that of cane sugar is $C_{12}H_{22}O_{11}$. By the addition of one molecule of water, H_2O, to a molecule of sucrose, two molecules of invert sugar (dextrose and glucose) are produced:[1] $C_{12}H_{22}O_{11} + H_2 = C_6H_{12}O_6 + C_6H_{12}O_6$. In bringing about this change, acids

are employed, but the acid in no way enters into the chemical composition of the final product; it is removed as described during the process of sugar manufacture. The action of the acid brings about a catalytic change, the acid being necessary only as a presence reagent to start the chemical reaction. When properly prepared and the acid product thoroughly removed, dextrose and glucose have practically the same food value as sugar. When they are digested, heat and energy are produced, and a given weight has about the same fuel value as an equal weight of sugar. Some of the glucose-yielding products can be made at less expense than sugar, and when they are sold under their right names there is no reason why they should not be used in the dietary, as they serve the same nutritive purpose.

79. Molasses is a by-product obtained in the refining of sugar. It is a mixture of cane sugar and invert sugars, as levulose and dextrose. When in sugar making the sucrose is removed by crystallization, a point is finally reached where the solution, or mother liquid, as it is called, refuses to give up any further crystals;[31] then this product, consisting of various sugars and small amounts of organic acids and ash, is partially refined and clarified to form molasses. The term "New Orleans" molasses was formerly applied to the product obtained by the use of open kettles for the manufacture of sugar, but during recent years the vacuum pan process has been introduced, and "New Orleans" molasses is now an entirely different article. The terms first, second, and third molasses are applied to the liquids obtained after the removal of the first, second, and third crops of sugar crystals; first molasses being richer in sucrose, while third molasses is richer in dextrose and invert sugars. The ash in molasses ranges from 4 to 6.5 per cent. Some of the low grades of molasses are used in the preparation of animal foods.

The taste and physical characteristics of molasses are due largely to the organic acids and impurities that are present, as well as to the proportion in which the various sugars occur. When used with soda in cooking and baking operations, the organic acid of the molasses liberates carbon dioxide gas, which acts as a leavening agent. Because of the organic acids, molasses should not be stored in tin or metalware dishes, as the solvent action results in producing poisonous tin and other metallic salts.

The food value of molasses is dependent entirely upon the amount of dry matter and the per cent of sugar. A large amount of water is considered an adulterant; ordinarily molasses contains from 20 to 33 per cent. If a sample of molasses contains 75 per cent of dry matter, it has slightly less than three fourths of the nutritive value of the same weight of sugar.

80. Syrups.--The term "syrup" is applied to natural products obtained by evaporation and purification of the saccharine juices of plants. Sorghum syrup is from the sorghum plant, which is pressed by machinery and the juice clarified and evaporated so as to contain about 25 per cent of water. In sorghum syrups there are from 30 to 45 per cent of cane sugar, and from 12 to 20 per cent of glucose and invert sugars. Cane syrup is made from the clarified juice of the sugar cane, and has about the same general composition as sorghum syrup. Maple syrup, prepared from the juice of the sugar maple, is characteristically rich in sucrose and contains but little glucose or reducing sugars. The flavor of all the syrups is due mainly to organic acids, ethereal products, and impurities. In some instances the essential flavor can be produced synthetically, or derived from other and cheaper materials; and by the use of these flavors, mixed syrups can be prepared closely resembling many of the natural products. When properly made, they are equal in nutritive value to natural syrups. When sold under assumed names, they are to be considered and classified as adulterated, and not as syrups from definite and specific products. Low-grade syrups and molasses are often used for making fuel alcohol. They readily undergo alcoholic fermentation and are valuable for this purpose, rendering it possible for a good grade of fuel alcohol to be produced at low cost. The manufacture of sugar, syrups, and molasses has been brought to a high degree of perfection through the assistance rendered by industrial chemistry. Losses in the process are reduced to a minimum, and the various steps are all controlled by chemical analysis. Sugar has the physical property of deflecting a ray of polarized light, the amount of deflection depending upon the quantity of sugar in solution. This is measured by the polariscope, an instrument by means of

which the sugar content of sugar plants is rapidly determined.

81. Honey is composed largely of invert sugars gathered by the honeybee from the nectar of flowers. It varies in composition and flavor according to its source. The color depends upon the flower from which it came, white clover giving a light-colored, pleasant-flavored honey, while that from buckwheat and goldenrod is dark and has a slightly rank taste. The comb is composed largely of wax, which has somewhat the same general composition as fat, but contains ethereal instead of glycerol bodies. On account of the predominance of invert sugars, pure honey has a levulo or left-handed rotation when examined by the polariscope. Honey contains from 60 to 75 per cent of invert sugars, and from 12 to 20 per cent of water, while the ash content is small, less than one tenth of one per cent. Strained honey is easily adulterated with glucose products. Adulteration with cane sugar is readily detected, as pure honey contains only a very small amount of sucrose. Honey can be made by feeding bees on sugar; the sugar undergoes inversion, with the production of dextrose. Such honey, although not adulterated, is inferior in quality and lacking in natural flavor.[18]

82. Confections.--By blending various saccharine products, confections are made. Usually sucrose (cane and beet sugar) is used as the basis for their preparation. Sucrose has definite physical properties, as crystalline structure, and forms chemical and mechanical combinations with acid, alkaline, and other substances; it also unites with water, and when heated undergoes changes in structural composition. The presence of small amounts of acid substances, or variations in the concentration of the sugar solution, materially affect the mechanical relation of the sugar particles to each other, and their crystallization. Usually crystallization takes place when there is less than 25 per cent of water present. The form, size, and arrangement of the crystals are influenced by agitation during cooling. To secure desired results, often small quantities of various other substances are employed for their mechanical action. Glucose is frequently used, and is said to be necessary for the production of some kinds of candy.

Candies are colored with various dyes and pigments, many of which are harmless, although some are injurious. Coal tar dyes are frequently employed for this purpose. Objection has generally been urged against their use, as it is believed many of them are injurious to health. It cannot be said, however, that all are poisonous, as some are known to be harmless. The use of a few coal tar dyes is allowed by the United States government. Mineral colors are now rarely, if ever, used.

Impure candies result from objectionable ingredients, as starch, paraffin, and large amounts of injurious coloring substances. Coal tar coloring materials are identified in the way described in Experiment No. 13. Confectionery, when properly prepared and unadulterated, has the same nutritive value as sugar and the other ingredients, and is entitled to a place in the dietary for the production of heat and energy. Much larger amounts of candies are sold and consumed during the winter than the summer months, suggesting that in cold weather candy is most needed in the dietary.

83. Saccharine is an artificial sweetening, five hundred times sweeter than cane sugar. It contains in its molecule, chemically united, benzine, sulphuric acid, and ammonia radicals. It is employed for sweetening purposes in cases of diabetes mellitus, where physicians advise against the use of sugar. It has no food value. A small amount is sometimes added to canned corn and tomatoes to impart a sweet taste. The physiological properties of saccharine have not been extensively investigated.

CHAPTER VI

LEGUMES AND NUTS

84. General Composition of Legumes.--Peas, beans, lentils, and peanuts are the legumes most generally used for human food. As a class, they are characterized by high protein content and a comparatively low per cent of starch and carbohydrates. They contain the largest amount of nitrogenous compounds of any of the vegetable foods, and hence are particularly

valuable in the human ration as a substitute for meats.[32] For feeding animals the legumes are highly prized, particularly the forage crops, clover and alfalfa. These secure their nitrogen, which is the characteristic element of protein, from the free nitrogen of the air, through the workings of bacterial organisms found in the nodules on the roots of the plants. The legumes appear to be the only plants capable of making use of the nitrogen of the air for food purposes.

85. Beans contain about 24 per cent of protein and but little fat, less than is found in any of the grain or cereal products. The protein of the bean differs from that of cereals in its general and structural composition. It is a globulin known as legumin, and is acted upon mainly by ferments working in alkaline solutions, as in the lower part of the digestive tract. Beans have about the same amount of ash as the cereals, but the ash is richer in potash and lime.

86. Digestibility of Beans.--Beans are usually considered indigestible, but experiments show they are quite completely digested, although they require more work on the part of the digestive tract than many other foods. The digestibility was found to vary with individuals, 86 per cent of the protein being digested in one case, and only 72 per cent in another. The protein of beans is not as completely digested as that of meats. When beans were combined with other foods, forming a part of a ration, they were more completely digested than when used in large amounts and with only a few other foods. The presence of the skin is in part responsible for low digestibility. When in the preparation of beans the skins, which contain a large amount of cellulose, are removed, the beans are more completely digested. By cooking from twenty minutes to half an hour in rapidly boiling water containing a small amount of soda, the skins are softened and loosened and are then easily removed by rubbing in cold water. Some of the soda enters into combination with the legumin. Along with the skins a portion of the germ is lost. The germ readily ferments, which is probably the cause of beans producing flatulence with some individuals during digestion. After the skins are removed the nutrients are more susceptible to the action of the digestive fluids. Experiments show that 42 per cent of the protein of baked

skinned beans is soluble in pepsin and pancreatin solutions, while under similar conditions there is only 3.85 per cent of the protein soluble from beans baked without removal of the skins.

87. Use of Beans in the Dietary.--There is no vegetable food capable of furnishing so much protein at such low cost as beans; from a pound costing five cents about one fifth of a pound of protein and three fifths of a pound of carbohydrates are obtained. Beans can, to a great extent, take the place of meats in the dietary. There is more protein in beans than in beef. Four ounces of uncooked beans or six ounces of baked beans are as much as can conveniently be combined in the dietary, and these will furnish a quarter of the protein of the ration. In the case of active out-of-door laborers over a pound of baked beans per day is often consumed with impunity.

88. String Beans.--String beans--green beans with pod--contain a large amount of water, 85 to 88 per cent. The dry matter is rich in protein, nearly 20 per cent, although in the green beans as eaten, containing 85 per cent water, there is less than 2-1/2 per cent. Lima beans are richer in protein than string beans, as the green pod is not included. String beans are valuable both for the nutrients they contain and for the favorable influence they exert upon the digestibility of other foods.

89. Peas.--In general composition and digestibility, peas are quite similar to beans. They belong to the same family, Leguminos? and the protein of each is similar in quantity and general properties. The statements made in regard to the composition, digestibility, and use of beans in the dietary apply with minor modifications to peas. When used in the preparation of soups, they add appreciable amounts of nutrients.

90. Canned Peas.--In order to impart a rich green color, copper sulphate has been used in the canning of peas. Physiologists differ as to its effect upon health. While a little may not be particularly injurious, much interferes with normal digestion of the food and forms insoluble copper proteids. In some countries a small amount of copper sulphate is tolerated, while in others it is

prohibited.

91. Peanuts.--Peanuts differ from peas and beans in containing more fat. They should be considered a food, for at ordinary prices they furnish a large amount of protein and fat. Like the other members of the legume family, the peanut is rather slow of digestion and requires considerable intestinal work for completion of the process.

NUTS

92. General Composition.--Nuts should be regarded as food, for they contribute to a ration appreciable amounts of nutrients. The edible portion of nearly all is rich in fat; pecans, for example, contain as high as 70 per cent. In protein content nuts range from 3 per cent in cocoanuts to 30 per cent in peanuts. The carbohydrate content is usually comparatively low, less than 5 per cent in hickory nuts, although there is nearly 40 per cent in chestnuts. On account of high fat content, nuts supply a large amount of heat and energy.[33]

93. Chestnuts are characterized by containing less fat and protein and much more carbohydrate material, especially starch, than is found in other nuts. In southern Europe chestnuts are widely used as food; the skins are removed, and the nuts are steamed, boiled, or roasted, and sometimes they are dried and ground into flour. Chestnuts are less concentrated in protein and fat, and form a better balanced food used alone than do other nuts.

94. The Hickory Nut, which is a characteristically American nut, contains in the edible portion about 15 per cent protein, 65 per cent fat, and 12 per cent carbohydrates.

95. The Almonds used in the United States come chiefly from southern Europe, although they are successfully raised in California. They contain about 55 per cent fat and 22 per cent protein. The flavor of almonds is due to a small amount of hydrocyanic acid.

96. Pistachio.--Some nuts are used for imparting color and flavor to food products, as the pistachio nut, the kernel of which is greenish in color and imparts a flavor suggestive of almonds. The pistachio has high food value, as it is rich in both fat and protein. It is employed in the manufacture of confectionery and in ice cream for imparting flavor and color.

97. Cocoanuts grow luxuriantly in many tropical countries, and have a high food value. They are characteristically rich in fat, one half of the edible portion being composed of this nutrient. For tropical countries they supply the fat of a ration at less expense than any other food. When used in large amounts they should be supplemented with foods rich in carbohydrates, as rice, and in proteids, as beans. Cocoanut milk is proportionally richer in carbohydrates and poorer in fat and protein than the meat of the cocoanut. In discussing the cocoanut, Woods states:[34]

"The small, green, and immature nuts are grated fine for medicinal use, and when mixed with the oil of the ripe nut it becomes a healing ointment. The jelly which lines the shell of the more mature nut furnishes a delicate and nutritious food. The milk in its center, when iced, is a most delicious luxury. Grated cocoanut forms a part of the world-renowned East India condiment, curry. Dried, shredded (desiccated) cocoanut is an important article of commerce. From the oil a butter is made, of a clear, whitish color, so rich in fat, that of water and foreign substances combined there are but O.0068. It is better adapted for cooking than for table use. At present it is chiefly used in hospitals, but it is rapidly finding its way to the tables of the poor, particularly as a substitute for oleomargarine."

98. Use of Nuts in the Dietary.--When nuts can be secured at a low price per pound, ten cents or less, they compare favorably in nutritive value with other staple foods. Digestion experiments with rations composed largely of nuts show that they are quite thoroughly digested. Professor Jaffa of the California Experiment Station, in discussing the nutritive value of nuts and fruits, says:[35]

"It is certainly an error to consider nuts merely as an accessory to an already heavy meal, and to regard fruit merely as something of value for its pleasant flavor, or for its hygienic or medicinal virtues. The agreement of one food or another with any person is more or less a personal idiosyncrasy, but it seems fair to say that those with whom nuts and fruits agree, can, if they desire, readily secure a considerable part of their nutritive material from such sources."

AVERAGE COMPOSITION OF NUTS

(From Fifteenth Annual Report, Maine Agricultural Experiment Station.)

==
======================= |REFUSE|EDIBLE | EDIBLE PORTION |VALUE[A] | | |-----------------------------| | |PORTION|Water|Prot.| Fat |Carb.| Ash | PER LB. --- ---------- | % | % | % | % | % | % | % |Calories Almonds | 64.8 | 35.2 | 1.7 | 7.3 |19.3 | 6.2 | 0.7 | 1065 Almonds, kernels | -- | 100.0 | 4.8 |21.0 |54.9 |17.3 | 2.0 | 3030 Brazil nuts | 49.6 | 50.4 | 2.7 | 8.6 |33.6 | 3.5 | 2.0 | 1545 Filberts | 52.1 | 47.9 | 1.8 | 7.5 |31.3 | 6.2 | 1.1 | 1575 Filberts, kernels | -- | 100.0 | 3.7 |15.6 |65.3 |13.0 | 2.4 | 3290 Hickory nuts | 62.2 | 37.8 | 1.4 | 5.8 |25.5 | 4.3 | 0.8 | 1265 Pecans | 49.7 | 50.3 | 1.4 | 5.2 |35.6 | 7.2 | 0.8 | 1733 Pecans, kernels | -- | 100.0 | 2.9 |10.3 |70.8 |14.3 | 1.7 | 3445 Walnuts | 58.0 | 42.0 | 1.2 | 7.0 |27.0 | 6.1 | 0.7 | 1385 Walnuts, kernels | -- | 100.0 | 2.8 |16.7 |64.4 |14.8 | 1.3 | 3305 Chestnuts | 16.1 | 83.9 |31.0 | 5.7 | 6.7 |39.0 | 1.5 | 1115 Acorns | 35.6 | 64.4 | 2.6 | 5.2 |24.1 |30.9 | 1.6 | 1690 Beechnuts | 40.8 | 59.2 | 2.3 |13.0 |34.0 | 7.8 | 2.1 | 1820 Butternuts | 86.4 | 13.6 | 0.6 | 3.8 | 8.3 | 0.5 | 0.4 | 430 Litchi nuts | 41.6 | 58.4 |10.5 | 1.7 | 0.1 |45.2 | 0.9 | 875 P. edulis | 40.6 | 59.4 | 2.0 | 8.7 |36.8 |10.2 | 1.7 | 1905   P. monophylla| 41.7 | 58.3 | 2.2 | 3.8 |35.4 |15.3 | 1.6 | 1850 P. sabiniana | 77.0 | 23.0 | 1.2 | 6.5 |12.3 | 1.9 | 1.1 | 675 Pistachio, kernels | -- | 100.0 | 4.2 |22.6 |54.5 |15.6 | 3.1 | 3010 Peanuts, raw | 26.4 | 73.6 | 6.9 |20.6 |30.7 |13.8 | 1.6 | 1935 Peanuts, kernels | -- | 100.0 | 9.3 |27.9 |42.0

|18.7 | 2.1 | 2640 Roasted peanuts | 32.6 | 67.4 | 1.1 |20.6 |33.1 |10.9 | 1.7 | 1985 Shelled peanuts | -- | 100.0 | 1.6 |30.5 |49.2 |16.2 | 2.5 | 2955 Peanut butter | -- | -- | 2.0 |29.3 |46.6 |17.1 |[B]5.0| 2830 Cocoanuts | 48.8 | 51.2 | 7.2 | 2.9 |25.9 |14.3 | 0.9 | 1415 Cocoanuts, shredded | -- | -- | 3.5 | 6.3 |57.3 |31.6| 1.3 | 3125 Cocoanut milk | -- | -- |92.7 | 0.4 | 1.5 | 4.6 | 0.8 | 97

===

====================

[Footnote A: Calculated from analyses.]

[Footnote B: Including salt, 4.1.]

CHAPTER VII

MILK AND DAIRY PRODUCTS

99. Importance in the Dietary.--There is no article of food which enters so extensively into the dietary as milk, and it is one of the few foods which supply all the nutrients,--fats, carbohydrates, and proteids.[36] Milk alone is capable of sustaining life for comparatively long periods, and it is the chief article of food during many diseases. An exclusive milk diet for a healthy adult, however, would be unsatisfactory; in the case of young children, milk is essential, because the digestive tract has not become functionally developed for the digestion of other foods.

It is necessary to consider not only the composition and nutritive value of milk, but also its purity or sanitary condition.

100. General Composition.--Average milk contains about 87 per cent water and 13 per cent dry matter. The dry matter is composed approximately of:

========================= | Per Cent Fat | 3.5 Casein | 3.25 Albumin | 0.50 Milk sugar | 5.00 Ash | 0.75 =========================

Fat is the most variable constituent of milk. Occasionally it is found as low as 2 per cent and as high as 6 per cent or more. The poorest and richest milks differ mainly in fat content, as the sugar, ash, casein, and albumin, or "solids of the milk serum," are fairly constant in amount and composition. Variations in the content of fat are due to differences in feed and in the breed and individuality of the animal.

101. Digestibility.--Milk is one of the most completely digested of foods, about 95 per cent of the protein and fat and 97 per cent of the carbohydrates being absorbed and utilized by the body.

In a mixed ration, the nutrients of milk are practically all absorbed. Milk also exerts a favorable influence upon the digestibility of other foods with which it is combined. This is doubtless due to the digestive action of the special ferments or enzymes which milk contains. In milk there is a soluble ferment material or enzyme which has the power of peptonizing proteids. It is this ferment which carries on the ripening process when cheese is cured in cold storage, and it is believed to be this body which promotes digestion of other foods with which milk is combined.[27]

Milk is not easily digested by some persons. The tendency to costiveness caused by a milk diet can be largely overcome by the use of salt with the milk, or of some solid food, as toast or crackers, to prevent coagulation and the formation of masses resistant to the digestive fluids. Barley water and lime water in small amounts are also useful for assisting mechanically in the digestion of milk. Milk at ordinary prices is one of the cheapest foods that can be used.

102. Sanitary Condition of Milk.--Equally as important as composition is the sanitary condition or wholesomeness of milk. Milk is a food material which readily undergoes fermentation and is a medium for the distribution of germ diseases. The conditions under which it is produced and the way in which it is handled determine largely its sanitary value, and are of so much importance in relation to public health that during recent years city and state

boards of health have introduced sanitary inspection and examination of milk along with the chemical tests for detecting its adulteration. Some of the more frequent causes of contaminated and unsound milk are: unhealthy animals, poor food and water, unsanitary surroundings of the animals, and lack of cleanliness and care in the handling and transporting of the milk. Outbreaks of typhoid and scarlet fevers and other germ diseases have frequently been traced to a contaminated milk supply.[37]

103. Certified Milk.--When milk is produced under the most sanitary conditions, the number of bacterial bodies per cubic centimeter is materially reduced. In order to supply high grade milk containing but few bacteria, special precautions are taken in the care of the animals, and in the feeding and milking, and all sources of contamination of the milk are eliminated as far as possible. Such milk, when sold in sterilized bottles, is commonly called "certified milk," indicating that its purity is guaranteed by the producer and that the number of bacteria per unit does not exceed a certain standard, as 8000 per cubic centimeter. Ordinary market milk contains upwards of 50,000.

104. Pasteurized Milk.--In order to destroy the activity of the bacterial organisms, milk is subjected to a temperature of 157?F. for ten minutes or longer, which process is known as pasteurization. When milk is heated to a temperature above 180? it is sterilized. Below 157? the albumin is not coagulated. By pasteurizing, milk is much improved from a sanitary point of view, and whenever the milk supply is of unknown purity, it should be pasteurized.[38] After the milk has been thus treated, the same care should be exercised in keeping it protected to prevent fresh inoculation or contamination, as though it were unpasteurized milk. For family use milk can be pasteurized in small amounts in the following way: Before receiving the milk, the receptacle should be thoroughly cleaned and sterilized with boiling water or dry heat, as in an oven. The milk is loosely covered and placed in a pan of water, a false bottom being in the pan so as to prevent unequal heating. The water surrounding the milk is gradually heated until a temperature of 159?F. is registered, and the milk is kept at this temperature

for about ten minutes. It is then cooled and placed in the refrigerator.

105. Tyrotoxicon.--Tyrotoxicon is a chemical compound produced by a ferment body which finds its way into milk when kept in unsanitary surroundings. It induces digestion disorders similar to cholera, and when present in large amounts, may prove fatal. It sometimes develops in cream, ice cream, or cheese, but only when they have been kept in unclean places or produced from infected milk.

601. Color of Milk is often taken as a guide to its purity and richness in fat. While a yellow tinge is usually characteristic of milks rich in fat, it is not a hard and fast rule, for frequently light-colored milks are richer in fat than yellow-tinged ones. The coloring material is independent of the percentage of fat, and it is not always safe to judge the richness of milk on the basis of color.

107. Souring of Milk.--Souring of milk is due to the action of the lactic acid organism, which finds its way into the milk through particles of dust carried in the air or from unclean receptacles which contain the spores of the organism.[39] When milk sours, a small amount of sugar is changed to lactic acid which reacts upon the casein, converting it from a soluble to an insoluble condition. When milk is exposed to the air at a temperature of from 70?to 90?F., lactic acid fermentation readily takes place. At a low temperature the process is checked, and at a high temperature the organisms and spores are destroyed. In addition to lactic acid ferments, there are large numbers of others which develop in milk, changing the different compounds of which milk is composed. In the processes of butter and cheese making, these fermentation changes are controlled so as to develop the flavor and secure the best grades of butter and cheese.

108. Use of Preservatives in Milk.--In order to check fermentation, boric acid, formalin, and other preservatives have been proposed. Physiologists object to their use because the quantity required to prevent fermentation is often sufficient to have a medicinal effect. The tendency is to use excessive

amounts, which may interfere with normal digestion of the food. Milk that is cared for under the most sanitary conditions has a higher dietetic value and is much to be preferred to that which has been kept sweet by the use of preservatives.

109. Condensed Milk is prepared by evaporating milk in vacuum pans until it is reduced about one fourth in bulk, when it is sealed in cans, and it will then keep sweet for a long time. Occasionally some cane sugar is added to the evaporated product. When diluted, evaporated milk has much the same composition as whole milk. When a can of condensed milk has been opened, the same care should be exercised to prevent fermentation as if it were fresh milk.

110. Skim Milk differs in composition from whole milk in fat content. When the fat is removed by the separator, there is often left less than one tenth of a per cent. Skim milk has a much higher nutritive value than is generally conceded, and wherever it can be procured at a reasonable price it should be used in the dietary as a source of protein.

111. Cream ranges in fat content from 15 to 35 per cent. It is generally preferred to whole milk, although it is not as well balanced a food, because it is deficient in protein. Cream should contain at least 25 per cent of fat.

112. Buttermilk is the product left after removal of the fat from cream by churning. It has about the same amount of nutrients as skim milk. The casein is in a slightly modified form due to the development of lactic acid during the ripening of the cream, and on this account buttermilk is more easily digested and assimilated by many individuals than milk in other forms. The development of the acid generally reduces the number of species of other than the lactic organisms, and these are increased.

113. Goat's Milk is somewhat richer in solids than cow's milk, containing about one per cent more proteids, a little more fat, and less sugar. When used as a substitute for human or cow's milk, it generally needs to be slightly

diluted, depending, however, upon the composition of the individual sample.

114. Koumiss is a fermented beverage made from milk by the use of yeast to secure alcoholic fermentation. Koumiss contains about one per cent each of lactic acid and alcohol, and the casein and other nutrients are somewhat modified by the fermentation changes. Koumiss is generally considered a non-alcoholic beverage possessing both food and dietetic value.

115. Prepared Milks.--Various preparations are made to resemble milk in general composition. These are mechanical mixtures of sugar, fats, and proteids. Milk sugar, casein, or malted proteids are generally the materials employed in their preparation. Often the dried and pulverized solids of skim milk are used. Many of the prepared milks are deficient in fat. While they are not equal to cow's milk, their use is often made necessary from force of circumstances.

116. Human Milk is not as rich in solid matter as cow's milk. It contains about the same amount of fat, one per cent more sugar, and one per cent less proteids. In human milk nearly one half of the protein is in the form of albumins, while in cow's milk there is about one fifth in this form. The fat globules are much smaller than those of cow's milk. In infant feeding it is often necessary to modify cow's milk by the addition of water, cream, and milk sugar, so as to make it more nearly resemble in composition human milk.

[Illustration: FIG. 25.--APPARATUS USED IN TESTING MILK.

1, pipette; 2, lactometer; 3, acid measure; 4, centrifuge; 5, test bottle.]

117. Adulteration of Milk.--Milk is not as extensively adulterated as it was before the passage and enforcement of the numerous state and municipal laws regulating its inspection and sale. The most frequent forms of adulteration are addition of water and removal of cream. These are readily detected from the specific gravity and fat content of the milk. The specific

gravity of milk is determined by means of the lactometer, an instrument which sinks to a definite point in pure milk. In watered milk it sinks to greater depth, depending upon the amount of water added. The fat content of milk is readily and accurately determined by the Babcock test, in which the fat is separated by centrifugal action. For the detection of adulterated milk the student is referred to Chapter VI, "Chemistry of Dairying," by Snyder.

BUTTER

118. Composition.--Butter is made by the churning or agitation of cream and is composed mainly of milk fats and water, together with smaller amounts of ash, salt, casein, milk sugar, and lactic acid. Average butter has the following composition:

	Per Cent
Water	10.5
Ash and salt	2.5
Casein and albumin	1.0
Fat	86.0

When butter contains an abnormal amount of water, it is considered adulterated. According to act of Congress standard butter should not contain over 16 per cent of water nor less than 82.5 per cent of fat.

119. Digestibility of Butter.--Digestion experiments show that practically all of the fat, 98 per cent, is digestible and available for use by the body. Butter is valuable only for the production of heat and energy. Alone, it is incapable of sustaining life, because it contains no proteid material. It is usually one of the more expensive items of food, but it is generally considered quite necessary in a ration.[5] It has been suggested that it takes an important part mechanically in the digestion of food.

120. Adulteration of Butter.--In addition to containing an excess of water, butter is adulterated in other ways. Old, stale butter is occasionally melted, washed, salted, and reworked. This product is known as renovated butter, and has poor keeping qualities. Frequently preservatives are added to such

butter to delay fermentation changes. Oleomargarine and butterine are made by mixing vegetable and animal fats.[40] Highly colored stearin, cotton-seed oil, and lard are the usual materials from which oleomargarine is made. It has practically the same composition, digestibility, and food value as butter. When sold under its true name and not as butter, there is no objection, as it is a valuable food and supplies heat and energy at less cost than butter. The main objection to oleomargarine and butterine is that they are sold as butter.[41]

The coloring of butter is not generally looked upon as adulteration, for butter naturally has a more or less yellow tinge. According to an act of Congress, butter colors of a non-injurious character are allowed to be used.

CHEESE

121. General Composition.--Cheese, is made by the addition of rennet to ripened milk, resulting in coagulation of the casein, which mechanically combines with the fat. It differs from butter in composition by containing, in addition to fat, casein and appreciable amounts of mineral matter. The composition varies with the character of the milk from which the cheese was made. Average milk produces cheese containing a larger amount of fat than proteids, while cheese from skimmed or partially skimmed milk is proportionally poorer in fat. Ordinarily there is about 35 per cent of water, 33 per cent of fat, and 27 per cent of casein, and albumin or milk proteids, the remainder being ash, salt, milk sugar, and lactic acid. Cheese is characterized by its large percentage of both fat and protein, and has high food value. It contains more fat and protein than any of the meats; in fact, there are but few foods which have such liberal amounts of these nutrients as cheese.

The odor and flavor of cheese are due to workings of bacteria which result in the production of aromatic compounds. The purity and condition of the milk, as well as the method of manufacture and the kind of ferment material used, determine largely the flavor and odor. Cheese is generally allowed to undergo a ripening or curing process before it is used as food. The changes resulting consist mainly in increased solubility of the proteids, with the formation of a small amount of amid and aromatic compounds.[42]

122. Digestibility.--Cheese is popularly considered an indigestible food, but extended experiments show that it is quite completely digested, although in the case of some individuals not easily digested. In general, about 95 per cent of the fat and 92 per cent and more of the protein is digested, depending upon the general composition of the cheese and the digestive capacity of the individual. As far as total digestibility is concerned, there appears to be but little difference between green and well-cured cheese. So far as ease of digestion is concerned, it is probable that some difference exists. There is also but little difference in digestibility resulting from the way in which milk is made into cheese, the nutrients of Roquefort, Swiss, Camembert, and Cheddar being about equally digestible.[13] The differences in odor and taste are due to variations in kind and amount of bacterial action. When combined with other foods, cheese may exercise a beneficial influence upon digestion in the same way as noted from the use of several foods in a ration. No material differences were observed in digestibility when cheese was used in small amounts, as for condimental purposes, or when used in large amounts to furnish nutrients. Artificial digestion experiments show that cheese is more readily acted upon by the pancreatic than by the gastric fluids, suggesting that cheese undergoes intestinal rather than gastric digestion. It is possible this is the reason that cheese is slow of digestion in the case of some individuals.

123. Use in the Dietary.--Cheese should be used in the dietary regularly and in reasonable amounts, rather than irregularly and then in large amounts. Cheese is not a luxury, but ordinarily it is one of the cheapest and most nutritious of human foods. A pound of cheese costing 15 cents contains about a quarter of a pound of protein and a third of a pound of fat; at the same price, beef yields only about half as much fat and less protein. Cheese at 18 cents per pound furnishes more available nutrients and energy than beef at 12 cents per pound. In the dietary of European armies, cheese to a

great extent takes the place of beef. See

Chapter XVI.

124. Cottage Cheese is made by coagulating milk and preparing the curd by mixing with it cream or melted butter and salt or sugar as desired. When milk can be procured at little cost, cottage cheese is one of the cheapest and most valuable foods.[43]

125. Different Kinds of Cheese.--By the use of different kinds of ferments and variations in the process of manufacture different types or kinds of cheese are made, as Roquefort, Swiss, Edam, Stilton, Camembert, etc. In the manufacture of Roquefort cheese, which is made from goats' and ewes' milk, bread is added and the cheese is cured in caves, resulting in the formation of a green mold which penetrates the cheese mass, and produces characteristic odor and flavor. Stilton is an English soft, rich cheese of mild flavor, made from milk to which cream is usually added. It is allowed to undergo an extended process of ripening, often resulting in the formation of bluish green threads of fungus. Limburger owes its characteristic odor and flavor to the action of special ferment bodies which carry on the ripening process. Neufchatel is a soft cheese made from sweet milk to which the rennet is added at a high temperature. After pressing, it is kneaded and worked, and then put into packages and covered with tin foil.

126. Adulteration of Cheese.--The most common forms of adulteration are the manufacture of skim-milk cheese by the removal of the fat from the milk, and substitution of cheaper and foreign fats, making a product known as filled cheese. When not labeled whole milk cheese, or sold as such, there is no objection to skim-milk cheese. It has a high food value and is often a cheap source of protein. The manufacture of filled cheese is now regulated by the national government, and all such cheese must pay a special tax and be properly labeled. As a result, the amount of filled cheese upon the market has very greatly decreased, and cheese is now less adulterated than in former years. The national dairy law allows the use of coloring matter of a harmless

nature in the manufacture of cheese.

127. Dairy Products in the Dietary.--The nutrients in milk are produced at less expense for grain and forage than the nutrients in beef, hence from a pecuniary point of view, dairy products, as milk and cheese, have the advantage. In the case of butter, however, the cost usually exceeds that of meat. In older agricultural regions, where the cost of beef production reaches the maximum, dairying is generally resorted to, as it yields larger financial returns, and as a result more cheese and less beef are used in the dietary. As the cost of meats is enhanced, dairy products, as cheese, naturally take their place.

CHAPTER VIII

MEATS AND ANIMAL FOOD PRODUCTS

128. General Composition.--Animal tissue is composed of the same classes of compounds as plant tissue. In each, water makes up a large portion of the weight, and the dry matter is composed of nitrogenous and non-nitrogenous compounds, and ash or mineral matter. Plants and animals differ in composition not so much as to the kinds of compounds, although there are differences, but more in the percentage amounts of these compounds. In plants, with the exception of the legumes, the protein rarely exceeds 14 per cent, and in many vegetable foods, when prepared for the table, there is less than 2 per cent. In meats the protein ranges from 15 to 20 per cent. The non-nitrogenous compounds of plants are present mainly in the form of starch, sugar, and cellulose, while in animal bodies there are only traces of carbohydrates, but large amounts of fat. Fat is the chief non-nitrogenous compound of meats; it ranges between quite wide limits, depending upon kind, age, and general condition of the animal. Meats contain the same general classes of proteins as the vegetable foods; in each the proteins are made up of albumins, glubulins, albuminates, peptone-like bodies, and insoluble proteids. The larger portion of the protein of meats and cereals is in insoluble forms. The meat juices, which contain the soluble portion of the

proteins, constitute less than 5 percent of the nitrogenous compounds. Meats contain less amid substances than plants, in which the amids are produced from ammonium compounds and are supposed to be intermediate products in the formation of proteids, while in the animal body they are derived from the proteids supplied in the food and, it is generally believed, cannot form proteids. Albuminoids make up the connective tissue, hair, and skin, and are more abundant in animal than in plant tissue. One of the chief albuminoids is gelatine. Both plant and animal foods undergo bacterial changes resulting in the production of alkaloidal bodies known as ptomaines, of which there are a large number. These are poisonous and are what cause putrid and stale meat to be unwholesome. The protein in meat differs little in general composition from that of vegetable origin; differences in structure and cleavage products between the two are, however, noticeable.

While meats from different kinds of animals have somewhat the same general composition, they differ in physical properties, and also in the nature of the various nutrients. For example, pork contains less protein than beef, but the protein of pork is materially different from that of beef, as a larger portion is in the form of soluble proteids, while in beef more is present in an insoluble form. Not only are differences in the percentage of individual proteins noticeable, but there are equally as great differences in the fats. As for example: some of the meats have a larger proportion of the fat as stearin than do others. Hence meats differ in texture and taste more than in nutritive value, due to the variations in the percentage of the different proteins, fats, and extractive material, rather than to differences in the total amounts of these compounds. The taste and flavor of meat is to a large extent influenced by the amount of extractive material.

While the nutrients of meats are divided into classes, as proteins and fats, there are a large number of separate compounds which make up each of the individual classes, and there are also small amounts of compounds which are not included in these groups.

129. Beef.--About one half of the weight of beef is water; the lean meat

contains a much larger amount than the fat. As a rule, the parts of the animal that contain the most fat contain the least water. In some meats there is considerable refuse, 25 to 30 per cent. In average meat about 12 per cent of the butcher's weight is refuse and non-edible parts.[44] A pound of average butcher's meat is about one half water, and over 10 per cent waste and refuse, which leaves less than 40 per cent fat and protein. Meat is generally considered to have a high nutritive value, due to the comparatively large amounts of fat and protein. Beef contains more protein than any vegetable food, except the legumes, and from 1 to 1.5 per cent mineral matter, exclusive of bone. Some of the mineral matter is chemically united with the protein and other compounds. While figures are given for average composition of beef, it is to be noted that wide variations are frequently to be met with, some samples containing a much larger amount of waste and trimmings than others, and this influences the percent of the nutritive substances. In making calculations of nutrients consumed, as in dietary studies, the figures for average composition of meat should be used only in cases where the samples do not contain an excess either of fat or trimmings.[45] When very lean, there is often a large amount of refuse, and the meat contains less dry matter and is of poorer flavor than from animals in prime condition. In the case of very fat animals, a large amount of waste results, and the flavor is sometimes impaired.

130. Veal differs from beef in containing a smaller amount of dry matter, richer in protein, but poorer in fat. Animals differ in composition at different stages of growth in much the same way as plants. In the earlier stages protein predominates in the plant tissue, while later the carbohydrates are added in larger amounts, reducing the percentage content of protein. In animals the same is noticeable. Young animals are, pound for pound, richer in protein than old animals. While in the case of vegetables the increase in size, or rotundity, is due to starch and carbohydrates, in animals it is due to the addition of fat. But plants, like animals, observe the same general laws as to changes in composition at different stages of growth.

131. Mutton.--There is about the same amount of refuse matter in mutton

as in beef. In a side of mutton about 19 percent: are trimmings and waste, and in a side of beef 18.5 per cent. Mutton, as a rule, contains a little more fat and dry matter than beef, and somewhat less protein. A side of beef, as purchased, contains about 50 per cent of water, 14.5 per cent protein, and 16.8 per cent of fat, while a side of mutton, as purchased, contains 42.9 per cent water, 12.5 per cent protein, and 24.7 per cent fat. A pound of beef yields a smaller number of calories by 25 per cent than a pound of mutton. At the same price per pound more nutrients can be purchased as mutton than as beef. The differences in composition between lamb and mutton are similar to those between veal and beef; viz. a larger amount of water and protein and a smaller amount of fat in the same weight of the young animals. Differences in composition between the various cuts of lamb are noticeable. The leg contains the least fat and the most protein, while the chuck is richest in fat and poorest in protein. As in the case of beef, many of the cheaper cuts contain as much or more nutrients than the more expensive cuts. They are not, however, as palatable and differ as to toughness and other physical characteristics.

132. Pork is characterized by a high per cent of fat and a comparatively low per cent of protein. It is generally richest in fat of any of the meats. The per cent of water varies with the fatness of the animal; in very fat animals there is a smaller amount, while lean animals contain more. In lean salt pork there is about 20 per cent water, and in fat salt pork about 7 per cent. There is less refuse and waste in pork than in either beef or mutton. Ham contains from 14 to 15 per cent of refuse, and bacon about 7 per cent. Bacon has nearly twice as much fat and a smaller amount of protein than ham. A pound of bacon, as purchased, will yield nearly twice as much energy or fuel value as a pound of ham. Digestion experiments show that bacon is quite readily and completely digested and is often a cheaper source of fat and protein than other meats. There is about three times as much fat in bacon as in beef. When prepared for the table bacon contains, from 40 to 50 per cent of fat. A pound of high grade, lean bacon furnishes from 0.1 to 0.3 of a pound of digestible protein and from 0.4 to 0.6 of a pound of digestible fat, which is about two thirds as much fat as is found in butter. Bacon contains nearly as

much digestible protein as other meats and from two to three times as much fat, making it, at the same price per pound, a cheaper food than other meats. In salt pork there is from 60 to 85 per cent of fat, and less protein than in bacon. The protein and fat of pork differ from those in beef not only in percentage amounts, but also in the nature of the individual proteins and fats. The composition of pork varies with the nature of the food that is consumed by the animal. Experiments show that it is possible by judicious feeding in the early stages of growth to produce pork with the maximum of lean meat and the minimum of fat. After the animal has passed a certain period, it is not possible by feeding to materially influence the percentage of nutrients in the meat. The flavor, too, of pork, as of other meats, is dependent largely upon the nature of the food the animal consumes. When there is a scant amount of available protein in the ration, the meat is dry, nearly tasteless, and contains less of the soluble nitrogenous compounds which impart flavor and individuality.

133. Lard is prepared from the fat of swine, and is separated from associated tissue by the action of heat. A large amount of fat is found lining the back of the abdominal cavity, and this is known as leaf lard. Slight differences are noticeable in the composition and quality of lard made from different parts of the hog. Leaf lard is usually considered the best. Lard is composed of the three fats, olein, stearin, and palmatin, and has a number of characteristic physical properties, as specific gravity, melting point, iodine absorption number, as well as behavior with various reagents, and these enable the mixing of other fats with lard to be readily detected. Lard is used in the preparation of oleomargarine, and it is also combined with various vegetable oils, as cotton-seed oil, in the making of imitation or compound lards.[46] Lard substitutes differ little in general composition from pure lard, except in the structure of the crystals and the percentage of the various individual fats.

134. Texture and Toughness of Meats.--In discussing the texture of meats, Professor Woods states:[45]

"Whether meats are tough or tender depends upon two things: the character of the walls of the muscle tubes and the character of the connective tissues which bind the tubes and muscles together. In young and well-nourished animals the tube walls are thin and delicate, and the connective tissue is small in amount. As the animals grow older or are made to work (and this is particularly true in the case of poorly nourished animals), the walls of the muscle tubes and the connective tissues become thick and hard. This is the reason why the flesh of young, well-fed animals is tender and easily masticated, while the flesh of old, hard-worked, or poorly fed animals is often so tough that prolonged boiling or roasting seems to have but little effect on it.

"After slaughtering, meats undergo marked changes in texture. These changes can be grouped under three classes or stages. In the first stage, when the meat is just slaughtered, the flesh is soft, juicy, and quite tender. In the next stage the flesh stiffens and the meat becomes hard and tough. This condition is known as rigor mortis, and continues until the third stage, when the first changes of decomposition set in. In hot climates the meat is commonly eaten in either the first or second stage. In cold climates it is seldom eaten before the second stage, and generally, in order to lessen the toughness, it is allowed to enter the third stage, when it becomes soft and tender, and acquires added flavor. The softening is due in part to the formation of lactic acid, which acts upon the connective tissue. The same effect may be produced, though more rapidly, by macerating the meat with weak vinegar. Meat is sometimes made tender by cutting the flesh into thin slices and pounding it across the cut ends until the fibers are broken."

135. Influence of Cooking upon the Composition of Meats.[47]--It is believed by many that losses are prevented and the nutritive value conserved when, in the cooking of meat, it is placed directly into boiling water rather than into cold water and then brought to the boiling point and cooked. Extensive experiments have been made by Dr. Grindley in regard to this and other points connected with the cooking of meats, and in general it was found that the temperature of the water in which the meat was placed made

little difference in its nutritive value or the amount of material extracted. It was found that by both methods there was dissolved 2.3 percent of the protein matter, 1 percent of the nitrogenous extractives, 1.6 per cent of non-nitrogenous material, and 0.8 per cent of ash, of the raw meat, which was equivalent to about 13 per cent of the total proteid material and 81 percent of the ash. The cold water extract contained bodies coagulated by heat. Cold water did not extract any of the fat, but during the process of cooking, appreciable amounts were lost mechanically. Cooked meats were found to be less soluble in cold water than raw meats. During the process of boiling, meat shrinks in weight about 40 or 45 per cent, depending mainly upon the size of the pieces and the content of fat. The loss in weight is practically a loss of water, and the loss of nutrients, all told, amounts to about 4 per cent, or more, depending upon the mechanical loss.[48] But slight differences were found in the composition of the meats cooked three and five hour periods.

"Careful study in this laboratory has shown that when meat is cooked in water at 80?to 85?C., placing meat in hot or cold water at the start has little effect on the amount of nutrients in the meat which passes into the broth. The meat was in the form of cubes, one to two inches, and in pieces weighing from one to two pounds.

"It is commonly supposed that when meat is plunged into boiling water, the albumin coagulates and forms a crust, which prevents the escape of nutritive materials into the broth. It is also believed that if a rich broth is desired, to be used either as a soup or with the meat as a stew, it is more desirable to place the meat in cold water at the start. From the results of these experiments, however, it is evident that, under these conditions, there can be little advantage in using hot or cold water at the beginning. When meats were cooked by dry heat, as in roasting, a larger amount of nutrients was rendered soluble in water than during boiling. The losses of nutrients were much smaller when meats were cooked by dry heat than when cooked in water, being on the average, water 35 per cent, nitrogenous extractives 9 per cent, non-nitrogenous extractives 17 per cent, fat 7 per cent, ash 12 per cent, and a small loss of protein."

The nutrients in the broth of the meat started in hot water amounted to about 1 per cent of protein, 1 per cent of fat, and O.5 per cent of ash, the amount of nutrients being directly proportional to the length of time and temperature of the cooking. In general, the larger the pieces, the smaller the losses. Beef that has been used in the preparation of beef tea loses its extractive materials, which impart taste and flavor, but there is only a small loss of actual nutritive value. Clear meat broth contains little nutriment--less than unfiltered broth. Most of the nitrogenous material of the broth is in the form of creatin, sarkin, and xanthin, nitrogenous extractives or amid substances having a much lower food value than proteids. Experiments show that some of these extractives have physiological properties slightly stimulating in their action, and it is believed the stimulating effect of a meat diet is in part due to these.[49] They are valuable principally for imparting taste and flavor, and cannot be regarded as nutrients. The variations in taste and flavor of meats from different sources are due largely to differences in extractive material.

"In general, the various methods of cooking materially modify the appearance, texture, and flavor of meat, and hence its palatability, but have little effect on total nutritive value. Whether it be cooked in hot water, as in boiling or stewing, or by dry heat, as in roasting, broiling, or frying, meat of all kinds has a high food value, when judged by the kind and amount of nutrient ingredients which are present." [50]

Beef extracts of commerce contain about 50 per cent of extractive matters, as amids, together with smaller amounts of soluble proteids; ash, mainly added salt, is also present in liberal amounts (20 per cent). Beef extracts have condimental value imparting taste and flavor, which make them useful for soup stocks, but they furnish little in the way of nutritive substance.

136. Miscellaneous Meat Products.--By combining different parts of the same animal, or different meats, a large number of products known as

sausage are made. These vary in composition with the ingredients used. In general, they are richer in fat than beef and contain about the same amount of protein. Potato flour and flour from cereals are sometimes used in their preparations, but the presence of any material amount, unless so stated on the package, is considered an adulterant.

Pickled meats are prepared by the use of condiments, as salt, sugar, vinegar, and saltpeter. During the smoking and curing of meats, no appreciable losses of nutrients occur.[51] The smoke acts as a preservative, and imparts condimental properties. Saltpeter (potassium nitrate) has been used from earliest times in the preparation of meats; it preserves color and delays fermentation changes. When used in moderate amounts it cannot be regarded as a preservative or injurious to health. Excessive amounts, however, are objectionable. Smoked meats, prepared with or without saltpeter, give appreciable reactions for nitrites, compounds formed during combustion of the wood by which the meat was smoked. Many vegetables contain naturally much larger amounts of nitrates, taken from the soil as food, than meat that has been preserved with saltpeter.[52]

137. Poultry.--The refuse and waste from chickens, as purchased on the market, ranges from 15 to 30 per cent. The fat content is much lower than in turkeys or ducks, the largest amount being found in geese. The edible portion of all fowls is rich in protein, particularly the dark meat, and the food value is about equal to that of meat in general. When it is desired to secure a large amount of protein with but little fat, chicken supplies this, perhaps, better than any other animal food. A difference is observed in the composition of the meat of young and old fowls similar to that between beef and veal. The physical composition and, to a slight extent, the solubility of the proteids are altered by prolonged cold storage, the difference being noticeable mainly in the appearance of the connective tissue of the muscles. In discussing poultry as food, Langworthy states:[53]

"A good, fresh bird shows a well-rounded form, with neat, compact legs, and no sharp, bony angles on the breast, indicating a lack of tender white meat. The skin should be a clear color (yellow being preferred in the American market) and free from blotches and pin feathers; if it looks tight and drawn, the bird has probably been scalded before being plucked. The flesh should be neither flabby nor stiff, but should give evenly and gently when pressed by the finger."

138. Fish.--From 30 to 60 per cent of the weight of fresh fish is refuse. The edible portion contains from 35 to 50 per cent, and in some cases more, of water. The dry matter is rich in protein; richer than many meats. The nutrients in fish range between comparatively wide limits, the protein in some cases being as low as 6 per cent, in flounder, and in others as high as 30 per cent, in dried codfish. The amount of fat, except in a few cases, as salmon and trout, is small. Salmon is the richest in fat of any of the fishes. When salted and preserved, the proportion of water is lessened and that of the nutrients is increased. Fish can take the place of meat in the dietary, but it is necessary to add a larger amount of fat to the ration because of the deficiency of most fish in this ingredient. Fish has about the same digestibility as meats. It is believed by many to be valuable because it supplies a large amount of available phosphates. Analyses, however, show that the flesh of fish contains no more phosphorus compounds than meats in general, and its food value is due to protein rather than to phosphates.[54]

Fish appears to be as completely and easily digested as meats. Differences in flavor, taste, and palatability are due to small amounts of flavors and extractive materials, varying according to the food consumed by the fish and the conditions under which they lived. The flesh of fish decays more readily than that of other meats and produces ptomaines, or toxic substances, which are the result of fermentation changes usually associated with putrefaction. Cases of poisoning from eating unsound fish are not infrequent.[55]

Shellfish have about the same general composition as fish. In clams there is a larger amount of dry matter than in oysters, which contain about 12 per cent, half of which is protein. When placed in fresh water, the oyster increases in size and undergoes the process known as "fattening."

Oftentimes impure water is used for this purpose, which makes the eating of raw oysters a questionable practice from a sanitary point of view, as the water in which they are floated often contains disease-producing germs, as typhoid. During the process of fattening, although the oyster increases in size and weight, it decreases in percentage of nutrients. In discussing the composition of oysters, Atwater states:[7]

"They come nearer to milk than almost any other food material as regards both the amounts and relative proportions of nutrients."

139. Eggs, General Composition.--Eggs are a type of concentrated nitrogenous food. About 75 per cent (shell removed) is water, about one third is yolk, and a little over 50 per cent is albumin or white. The shell makes up from 10 to 12 per cent of the weight. The yolk and white differ widely in composition. The yolk contains a much larger per cent of solids than the white, and is rich in both fat and protein, from a third to a half of the weight being fat. The white has about the same amount of water, 88 per cent, as average milk, but, unlike milk, the dry matter is mainly albumin. The entire egg (edible portion) contains about equal parts of fat and protein; 12 to 13 per cent of each and an appreciably large amount of ash or mineral matter,--from 0.8 to 1 per cent, consisting mainly of phosphates associated with the albumin. There is no material difference in chemical composition between white and dark shelled eggs, or between eggs with different colored yolks. It is simply a question of coloring matter. The egg is influenced to an appreciable extent by feed and general care of the fowls. The egg and the potato contain about the same amount of water. They are, however, distinct types of food, the potato being largely composed of carbohydrates and the egg of protein and fat. Eggs resemble meat somewhat in general composition, although they contain rather less of protein and fat. When eggs are boiled there is a loss of weight due to elimination of water; otherwise the composition is unaltered, the coagulation of the albumin, as stated in Chapter I, consisting simply in a rearrangement of the atoms of the molecule. The egg is particularly valuable in the dietary of the convalescent, when it is desired to secure the maximum amount of phosphorus in organic

combination.

The flavor of eggs is in part due to the food supplied to the fowls, as well as the age of the egg. Experiments show that onions and some other vegetables, when fed to fowls, impart odors and taste to the eggs. The keeping qualities of eggs are also dependent upon the food supplied. In experiments at the Cornell Experiment Station, when hens were fed on a narrow, nitrogenous ration, a large number of eggs were produced containing the minimum amount of solid matter and of poor keeping quality, while a larger sized egg of better keeping quality was obtained when a variety of foods, nitrogenous and non-nitrogenous, was supplied.

140. Digestibility of Eggs.--Digestion experiments show that there is but little difference in the digestibility of eggs cooked in different ways. A noticeable difference, however, is observed in the rapidity with which the albumin and proteids are dissolved in a pepsin solution. In general, it was found that, when the albumin was coagulated at a temperature of 180? it was more rapidly and completely dissolved in the pepsin than when coagulated at a temperature of 212? When eggs were cooked at a temperature of 212? the hard-boiled eggs appeared to be slightly more digestible than the soft-boiled eggs, but the digestion was not as complete as when the cooking was done at a temperature of 180? then no difference in digestibility was found between eggs cooked for a short or a long time. The egg is one of the most completely digested of all foods, practically all the protein and fat being absorbed and available to the body. Langworthy, in discussing Jorissenne's investigations on the digestibility of eggs, states:[53]

"The yolk of raw, soft-boiled, and hard-boiled eggs is equally digestible. The white of soft-boiled eggs, being semi-liquid, offers little more resistance to the digestive juices than raw white. The white of a hard-boiled egg is not generally very thoroughly masticated. Unless finely divided, it offers more resistance to the digestive juices than the fluid or semi-fluid white, and undigested particles may remain in the digestive tract many days and decompose. From this deduction it is obvious that thorough mastication is a matter of importance. Provided mastication is thorough, marked differences in the completeness of digestion of the three sorts of eggs, in the opinion of the writer cited, will not be found."

141. Use of Eggs in the Dietary.--When eggs are at the same price per dozen as meat is per pound, they furnish a larger amount of nutrients. In general, a dozen eggs have a little higher food value than a pound of meat. Eggs are usually a cheaper source of food because a smaller amount is served than of meat. When eggs are 25 cents per dozen, the cost of ten eggs for a family of five is less than that of a pound or a pound and a quarter of beef at 22 cents per pound. The meat, however, would furnish the larger amount of nutrients. Eggs are valuable, too, in the dietary because they are frequently combined with flour, cereal products, and vegetables, which contain a large amount of starch, and some of which contain small amounts of protein. This combination furnishes a balanced ration, as well as secures palatability and good mechanical combination of the foods. Eggs in combination with flour, sugar, butter, and other materials have equally as great a value as when used alone and as a substitute for meat.

Eggs vary in weight from 17.5 to 28 ounces, and more per dozen. They should be purchased and sold by weight. When stored, eggs lose weight. The egg cannot be considered as entirely germ proof, and care is necessary in its handling and use, the same as with other food articles. The cause of the spoiling of eggs is due largely to exterior bacterial infection.

CANNED MEATS

142. General Composition.--Canned meats differ but little in composition from fresh meats. Usually during the process of cooking and canning there is a slight increase in the amount of dry matter, but the relative proportion of protein and fat is about the same as in fresh meat. It is frequently stated that the less salable parts are used in the preparation of canned meats, as it is possible by cooking and the addition of condiments to conceal the inferior physical properties. As to the accuracy of these statements, the author is

unable to say. The shrinkage or loss in weight during canning amounts to from 30 to 40 per cent. The liquids in which the cooking and parboiling are done are sometimes used in the preparation of beef extracts. Salt, saltpeter, and condiments are generally added during the canning process. Saltpeter is used, as it assists in retaining the natural color and prevents some objectionable fermentation changes. In moderate amounts it is not generally considered an adulterant. An extensive examination by Wiley and Bigelow of packing-house products and preserved meats showed that of the latter only a small amount contained objectionable preservatives. The authors, after an extended investigation, reported favorably upon their composition and sanitary value, saying they found "so little to criticise and so much to commend in these necessary products." In this bulletin they do not classify saltpeter as an adulterant.[51]

Where fresh meats cannot be secured, canned meats are often indispensable. Usually the nutrients of canned meats cost more than those of fresh meats, and in their use as food much care should be exercised to prevent contamination after opening the cans. Occasionally the meat contains ferment materials that have not been entirely destroyed during cooking, and these, when the cans are stored in warm places, develop and cause deleterious changes to occur. Consequently canned meats should be stored at a low temperature. By recent congressional act, these preparations are now made under the supervision of government inspectors. All diseased animals are rejected, and the sanitary conditions under which the meat is prepared have been greatly improved. Formerly, the most frequent forms of adulteration were substitution of one meat for another, as the mixing of veal with chicken, and the use of preservatives, as borax and sulphites. While the cost of the nutrients in canned meats is generally much higher than in fresh meats, the latter are not always easily obtained, or capable of being kept for any length of time, and hence canned meats are often indispensable.

CHAPTER IX

CEREALS

143. Preparation and Cost of Cereals.--The grains used in the preparation of cereal foods are wheat, oats, corn, rice, and, to a less extent, barley and rye. For some of these the entire cleaned grain is ground or pulverized, while for others the bran and germ are first removed. In order to improve their keeping qualities, they are often sterilized before being put up in sealed packages. Special treatment, as steaming or malting, is sometimes given to impart palatability and to lessen the time required for cooking. As a class, the cereal foods are clean, nutritious, and free from adulteration. Extravagant claims are sometimes made as to their food value, and frequently excessive prices are charged, out of proportion to the cost of the nutrients in the raw material. Within recent years the number of cereal preparations has greatly increased, due to improvements and variations in the methods of manufacture.[56]

Cereal foods are less expensive than meats and the various animal food products. They contain no refuse, are easily prepared for the table, and may be kept without appreciable deterioration. Some of the ready--to-eat brands are cooked, dried, and crushed, and sugar, glucose, salt, and various condimental materials added to impart taste. Others contain malt, or are subjected to a malting or germinating process to develop the soluble carbohydrates, and such foods are sometimes called predigested. It is believed that the cereals are being more extensively used in the dietary, which is desirable both from an economic and a nutritive point of view. Special care is necessary in the cooking and preparation of cereals for the table, in order to develop flavor and bring about hydration and rupturing of the tissues, as explained in Chapter II.

144. Corn Preparations.--Corn or maize is characterized by a high percent of fat and starch, and, compared with wheat and oats, a low content of protein.[57] Removal of the bran and germ lessens the per cent of fat. The germ is removed principally because it imparts poor keeping qualities. Many of the corn breakfast foods contain 1 per cent or less of fat and from 8 to 9 per cent of protein. Coarsely ground corn foods are not as completely digested and assimilated as those more finely ground. As in the case of

wheat products, the presence of the bran and germ appears to prevent the more complete absorption of the nutrients. Finely ground corn meal compares favorably in digestibility with wheat flour. Corn flour is prepared by removal of the bran and germ and granulation of the more starchy portions of the kernel, and has better keeping qualities than corn meal from which the bran and germ have not been so completely removed. At times corn flour has been sufficiently low in price to permit its use for the adulteration of wheat flour. The mixing of corn and wheat flours, however, is prohibited by law unless the product is so labeled. When combined with wheat flour, corn bread and various other articles of food are prepared, but used alone corn flour is not suitable for bread making, because its gluten lacks the binding properties imparted to wheat flour by the gliadin. It is essential that corn be used with foods of high protein content so as to make a balanced ration; for when it forms a large part of the dietary, the ration is apt to be deficient in protein. In a mixed dietary, corn is one of the cheapest and best cereals that can be used. Too frequently, however, excessive prices are charged for corn preparations that contain no more nutrients than ordinary corn meal. There is no difference between yellow and white corn meal so far as nutritive value is concerned.

145. Oat Preparations are characterized by large amounts of both protein and fat. Because of the removal of the hulls, they contain more protein than the original grain. The oat preparations differ little in chemical composition. They all have about 16 per cent of protein, 7 per cent of fat, and 65 per cent of starch, and are richer in ash or mineral matter than other cereals. The main difference is in method of preparation and mechanical composition. Some are partially cooked and then dried. Those costing 7 cents or more per pound do not contain any greater amount of nutritive substance than those purchased in bulk at about half the price. At one time it was believed that oats contained a special alkaloid having a stimulating effect when fed to animals. Recent investigations, however, show that there is no alkaloidal material in oats, and whatever stimulating effect they may have results from the nutrients they contain. Occasionally there is an appreciable amount of cellulose, or fiber, left in the oat preparations, due to imperfect milling. This

noticeably lowers the digestibility. Oatmeal requires much longer and more thorough cooking than many other cereals, and it is frequently used as food when not well prepared. Digestion experiments show that when oatmeal is cooked for four hours or more, it is more readily acted upon by the diastase ferment and digested in a shorter time than oatmeal cooked only a half hour.[5] Oatmeal is one of the cheapest sources from which protein is obtained, and when well cooked it can advantageously form an essential part of the ration. Unless thoroughly cooked, the oat preparations do not appear to be quite so completely or easily digested as some of the other cereals.

146. Wheat Preparations differ in chemical composition more than those from oats or corn, because wheat is prepared in a greater variety of ways. They are made either from the entire kernel, including the bran and germ, or from special parts, as the granular middlings, as in the case of some of the breakfast foods, and a few are made into a dough and baked, then dried and toasted. Some special flours are advertised as composed largely of gluten, but only those that have been prepared by washing out the starch are entitled to be classed as gluten flours.[58] For the food of persons suffering from diabetes mellitus physicians advise the use of flour low in starch, and this can be made by washing and thus removing a portion of the starch from wheat flour, as directed in Experiment No. 30. The glutinous residue is then used for preparing articles of food. Analyses of some of the so-called gluten flours show that they contain no more gluten than ordinary flour, particularly the low grades. A number of wheat breakfast foods are prepared by sterilizing the flour middlings obtained after removal of the bran and germ. These middlings are the same stock or material from which the patent grades of flour are made, and they differ from wheat flour only in mechanical structure and size of the particles. Where granular wheat middlings can be secured in bulk at the same price as flour they furnish a valuable and cheap cereal breakfast food.

As to the digestibility and food value, the wheat breakfast foods have practically the same as graham, entire wheat, or ordinary patent flour, depending upon the stock which they contain. Those with large amounts of bran and germ are not as completely digested as when these parts of the kernel are not included. Wheat preparations, next to oats, have the most protein of any of the cereal foods. Occasionally they are prepared from wheats low in gluten and not suitable for bread-making purposes. When purchased in bulk the wheat preparations are among the cheapest foods that can be used in the dietary.[56]

147. Barley Preparations are not so extensively used as wheat, oats, and corn. Barley contains a little more protein than corn, but not quite so much as wheat; otherwise it is quite similar to wheat in general composition. Sometimes in the preparation of breakfast foods barley meal is mixed with wheat or corn. Barley is supposed to be more readily digested than some of the other cereals, because of the presence of larger amounts of active ferment bodies, and it is frequently used for making an extract known as "barley water," which, although it contains very little nutritive value, as less than one per cent of the weight of the barley is rendered soluble, is useful in its soothing influence and mechanical action upon the mucous membrane of the digestive tract.

148. Rice Preparations.--Rice varies somewhat in composition, but usually contains a slightly lower percentage of protein than corn and also a smaller amount of fat. It is particularly rich in starch, and has the least ash or mineral matter of any of the cereals. In order to make a balanced ration, rice should be supplemented with legumes and other foods rich in proteids. It is a valuable grain, but when used alone it is deficient in protein. Rice is digested with moderate ease, but is not as completely absorbed by the body as other cereals, particularly those prepared by fine grinding or pulverization. Of late years rice culture has been extensively introduced into some of the southern states, and the domestic rice seems to have slightly higher protein content than the imported. Rice contains less protein than other cereals, and the starch grain is of different construction. Rice does not require such prolonged cooking as oatmeal; it needs, however, to be thoroughly cooked.

149. Predigested Foods.[56]

"It is questionable whether it would be of advantage to a healthy person to have his food artificially digested. The body under normal conditions is well adapted to utilize such foods as the ordinary mixed diet provides, among them the carbohydrates from the cereals. Moreover, it is generally believed that for the digestive organs, as for all others of the body, the amount of exercise they are normally fitted to perform is an advantage rather than the reverse. It has been said that 'a well man has no more need of predigested food than a sound man has for crutches.' If the digestive organs are out of order, it may be well to save them work, but troubles of digestion are often very complicated affairs, and the average person rarely has the knowledge needed to prescribe for himself. In general, those who are well should do their own work of digestion, and those who are ill should consult a competent physician."--WOODS AND SNYDER.

150. The Value of Cereals in the Dietary.--Cereals are valuable in the dietary because of the starch and protein they supply, and the heat and energy they yield. They are among the most inexpensive of foods and, when properly prepared, have a high degree of palatability; then, too, they are capable of being blended in various ways with other foods. Some are valuable for their mechanical action in digestion, rather than for any large amount of nutrients. They do not furnish the quantity of mineral matter and valuable phosphates that is popularly supposed. They all contain from 0.5 to 1.5 percent of mineral matter, of which about one third is phosphoric anhydrid. In discussing the phosphate content of food, Hammersten states:[59]

"Very little is known in regard to the need of phosphates or phosphoric acid.... The extent of this need is most difficult to determine, as the body shows a strong tendency, when increased amounts of phosphorus are introduced, to retain more than is necessary. The need of phosphates is relatively smaller in adults than in young developing animals."

In the coarser cereals, which include the bran and germ, there is the maximum amount of mineral matter, but, as in the case of graham bread, it is not as completely digested and absorbed by the body as the more finely granulated products which contain less. The kind of cereal to use in the dietary is largely a matter of personal choice. As only a small amount is usually eaten at a meal, there is little difference in the quantity of nutrients supplied by the various breakfast cereals.

TOTAL AND DIGESTIBLE NUTRIENTS AND FUEL VALUE OF CEREALS [Transcriber's note: This table has been divided into two parts to fit limits on page width.]

```
================================================================
= | TOTAL NUTRIENTS | |-----+----+----+----------+----+ | | | | C.H. | | KIND
OF FOOD |Water|Pro.|Fat +----+-----+Ash | | | | |N.F.|Fiber| | | | |Ext | | | ------
----------------+-----+----+----+----+-----+----+ | % | % | % | % | % | % | Oat
Preparations: | | | | | | | Oats, whole grain | 11.0|11.8| 5.0|59.7| 9.5| 3.0|
Oatmeal, raw | 7.3|16.1| 7.2|66.6| 9.9| 1.9| Rolled, steam-cooked| 8.2|16.1|
7.4|65.2| 1.3| 1.8| Wheat: | | | | | | | Whole grain | 10.5|11.9| 2.1|71.9| 1.8| 1.8|
Cracked wheat | 10.1|11.1| 1.7|73.8| 1.7| 1.6| Rolled, steam-cooked|
10.6|10.2| 1.8|74.4| 1.8| 1.5| Shredded wheat | 8.1|10.6| 1.4|76.6| 2.1| 1.8|
Crumbed and malted | 5.6|12.2| 1.0|77.6| 1.7| 1.0| Farina | 10.9|11.0| 1.4|75.9|
0.4| 0.4| Rye: | | | | | | | Whole grain | 11.6|10.6| 1.7|72.5| 1.7| 1.9| Flaked, to be
eaten | 11.1|10.0| 1.4| 75.8 | 1.7| raw | | | | | | | Barley: | | | | | | | Whole grain |
10.9|12.4| 1.8|69.8| 2.7| 2.4| Pearled barley | 11.5| 8.5| 1.1|77.5| 0.3| 1.1|
Buckwheat: | | | | | | | Flour | 13.6| 6.4| 1.2|77.5| 0.4| 0.9| Corn: | | | | | | | Whole
grain | 10.9|10.5| 5.4|69.6| 2.1| 1.5| Corn meal, unbolted | 11.6| 8.4| 4.7| 74.0 |
1.3| Corn meal, bolted | 12.5| 9.2| 1.9|74.4| 1.0| 1.0| Hominy | 10.9| 8.6|
0.6|79.2| 0.4| 0.3| Pop corn, popped | 4.3|10.7| 5.0|77.3| 1.4| 1.3| Hulled corn |
74.1| 2.3| 0.9| 22.2 | 0.5| Rice: | | | | | | | Whole rice, polished| 12.3| 6.9| 0.3|
80.0 | 0.5| Puffed rice | 7.1| 6.2| 0.6| 85.7 | 0.4| Crackers | 6.8|10.7| 8.8|71.4|
0.5|    1.8|    Macaroni    |    10.3|13.4|    0.9|    74.1    |    1.3|
================================================================
=
```

KIND OF FOOD	Pro.	Fat	C.H.	Ash	Fuel Value per lb. Calories.
	%	%	%	%	
Oat Preparations:					
Oats, whole grain	--	--	--	--	--
Oatmeal, raw	12.5	6.5	65.5	1.4	1767
Rolled, steam-cooked	12.5	6.7	64.5	1.4	1759
Wheat:					
Whole grain	--	--	--	--	--
Cracked wheat	8.1	1.5	68.7	1.2	1501
Rolled, steam-cooked	8.5	1.6	70.7	1.1	1541
Shredded wheat	7.7	1.3	71.1	1.4	1521
Crumbed and malted	9.1	0.9	73.7	1.4	1623
Farina	8.9	1.3	72.9	0.5	1609
Rye:					
Whole grain	--	--	--	--	--
Flaked, to be eaten	7.8	1.3	71.1	1.3	1516
raw					
Barley:					
Whole grain	--	--	--	--	--
Pearled barley	6.6	1.0	73.0	0.3	1514
Buckwheat:					
Flour	5.0	1.1	73.1	0.7	1471
Corn:					
Whole grain	--	--	--	--	--
Corn meal, unbolted	6.2	4.2	73.2	1.0	1728
Corn meal, bolted	6.8	1.7	74.6	0.8	1602
Hominy	6.4	0.5	78.7	0.2	1671
Pop corn, popped	7.9	4.5	77.8	1.0	1882
Hulled corn	1.7	0.8	21.8	0.4	492
Rice:					
Whole rice, polished	5.8	0.3	78.4	0.4	1546
Puffed rice	5.1	0.5	84.0	0.3	1639
Crackers	9.1	7.9	70.5	1.4	1905
Macaroni	11.6	0.8	72.2	1.0	1660

CHAPTER X

WHEAT FLOUR

151. Use for Bread Making.--Wheat is particularly adapted to bread-making purposes because of the physical properties of the gliadin, one of its proteids. It is the gliadin which, when wet, binds together the flour particles, enabling the gas generated during bread making to be retained, and the loaf to expand and become porous. Wheat varies in chemical composition between wide limits; it may contain as high as 16 per cent of protein, or as low as 8 per cent; average wheat has from 12 to 14 per cent; and with these differences in composition, the bread-making value varies.

152. Winter and Spring Wheat Flours.--There are two general classes of wheat: spring wheat and winter wheat. The winter varieties are seeded in the fall, and the spring varieties, which are grown mainly in the Northwestern states, Minnesota, and North and South Dakota, and the Canadian Northwest, are seeded in the spring and mature in the late summer. Winter wheat is confined to more southern latitudes and regions of less severe winter, and matures in the early summer. There are many varieties of both spring and winter wheat, although wheats are popularly characterized only as hard or soft, depending upon the physical properties. The winter wheats are, as a rule, more soft and starchy than the spring wheats, which are usually corneous or flinty to different degrees. There is a general tendency for wheats to become either starchy or glutinous, owing to inherited individuality of the seed and to environment. There are often found in the same field wheat plants yielding hard glutinous kernels, and other plants producing starchy kernels containing 5 per cent less proteids. Wheats of low protein content do not make high-grade flour; neither do wheats of the maximum protein content necessarily make the best flour. For a more extended discussion of wheat proteids, the student is referred to

Chapter XI.

153. Composition of Wheat and Flour.--In addition to 12 to 14 per cent proteids, wheat contains 72 to 76 per cent of starch and small amounts of other carbohydrates, as sucrose, dextrose, and invert sugar. The ash or mineral matter ranges from 1.7 to 2.3 per cent. There is also about 2 per cent fiber, 2.25 per cent ether extract or crude fat, and about 0.2 per cent organic acids.

Summary:

COMPOSITION OF WHEAT FLOUR

==

== | Per Cent Water | 12.00 | {Potash } | {Soda } | {Lime } | Ash {Magnesia }
| 2.25 {Phosphoric anhydrid} | {Sulphuric anhydrid } | {Other substances } |
| {Albumin 0.4} | {Globulin 0.9} | Protein {Gliadin 6.0} | 13.00 {Glutenin
5.3} | {Other proteids 0.4} | Other nitrogenous bodies, as amids, lecethin |
0.25 Crude fat, ether extract | 2.25 Cellulose | 2.25 Starch | 66.00 Sucrose,
dextrose, soluble carbohydrates, etc.| 2.00

==
=

154. Roller Process of Flour Milling.--Flours vary in composition, food
value, and bread-making qualities with the character of the wheat and the
process of milling employed. Prior to 1870 practically all wheat flour was
prepared by grinding the wheat between millstones; but with the
introduction of the roller process, steel rolls were substituted for
millstones.[60] By the former process a smaller amount of flour was secured
from the wheat, but with the present improved systems about 75 per cent of
the weight of the grain is recovered as merchantable flour and 25 per cent as
wheat offals, bran, and shorts[61].

The wheat is first screened and cleaned, then passed on to the corrugated
rolls, or the first break, where it is partially flattened and slightly crushed
and a small amount of flour, known as the break flour, is separated by means
of sieves, while the main portion is conveyed through elevators to the second
break, where the kernels are more completely flattened and the granular
flour particles are partially separated from the bran. The material passes over
several pairs of rolls or breaks, each succeeding pair being set a little nearer
together. This is called the gradual reduction process, because the wheat is
not made into flour in one operation. More complete removal of the bran and
other impurities from the middlings is effected by means of sieves,
aspirators, and other devices, and the purified middlings are then passed on
to smooth rolls, where the granulation is completed. The flour finally passes
through silk bolting cloths, containing upwards of 12,000 meshes per square
inch. The dust and fine debris particles are removed at various points in the
process. The granulation of the middlings is done after the impurities are

removed, the object being first to separate as perfectly as possible the middlings from the branny portions of the kernel. If the wheat were first ground into a fine meal, it would be impossible to secure complete separation of the flour from the offal portions of the kernel.

Flour milling is entirely a mechanical process; the flour stock passes from roll to roll by means of elevators. According to the number of reductions which the middlings and stock undergo, the milling is designated as a long or a short reduction system; the term 4, 6, 8, or 10 break process means that the stock has been subjected to that number of reductions. With an 8-break system of milling, the process is more gradual than with a 4-break, and greater opportunity is afforded for complete removal of the bran. In some large flour mills, the wheat is separated into forty or more different products, or streams, as they are called, so as to secure a better granulation and more complete removal of the offals, after which many of these streams are brought together to form the finished flour. What is known as patent flour is derived from the reduction of the middlings, while the break flours are recovered before the offals are completely removed; hence they are not of so high a grade. No absolute definition can be given, however, of the term "patent flour," as usage varies the meaning in different parts of the country.

155. Grades of Flour.--Flour is the purified, refined, and bolted product obtained by reduction and granulation of wheat during and after the removal of the branny portions of the wheat kernel. It is defined by proclamation of the Secretary of Agriculture, under authority of an act of Congress, as: "Flour is the fine, sound product made by bolting wheat meal, and contains not more than thirteen and one half (13.5) per cent of moisture, not less than one and twenty-five hundredths (1.25) per cent of nitrogen, not more than one (1) per cent of ash, and not more than fifty hundredths (0.50) per cent of fiber."

Generally speaking, flour may be divided into two classes, high grade and low grade. To the first class belong the first and second patents and, according to some authorities, a portion of the straight grade, or standard patent flour, and to the second class belong the second clear and "red dog." About 72 per cent of the cleaned wheat as milled is recovered in the higher grades of flour, and about 2 or 3 per cent as low grades, a large portion of which is sold as animal food. The high grades are characterized by a lighter color, more elastic gluten, better granulation, and a smaller number of debris particles. Although the lower grade flours contain a somewhat higher percentage of protein, they are not as valuable for bread-making purposes because the gluten is not as elastic, and consequently they do not make as good bread. If the impurities from the low grades could be further eliminated, it is believed that less difference would exist between high and low grade flours.

Various trade names are used to designate flours, as a 95 per cent patent, meaning that 95 per cent of the total flour is included in the patent; or an 85 per cent patent, when 85 per cent of all the flour is included in that particular patent. If all the flour streams were purified and blended, and only one grade of flour made, it would be called a 100 per cent patent. An 85 per cent patent is a higher grade flour than a 95 per cent patent.

156. Composition of Flour.--The composition of the different grades of flour made from the same wheat is given in the following table:[62]

COMPOSITION, ACIDITY, AND HEATS OF COMBUSTION OF FLOURS AND OTHER MILLED PRODUCTS OF WHEAT

```
===============================================================
======================= |WATER| PROTEIN | FAT| CARBO-| ASH|
ACIDITY | HEAT OF MILLED PRODUCT | |(N ?5.7)| | HY- | | CALCUL-
|COMBUSTION | | | | DRATES| |ATED AS | PER GRAM | | | | | |LACTIC
|DETERMINED | | | | | | ACID | ----------------------------------------------------------
---------------------- | % | % | % | % | % | % |Calories First patent flour |10.55|
11.08 |1.15| 76.85 |0.37| 0.08 | 4032 Second patent flour |10.49| 11.14 |1.20|
76.75 |0.42| 0.08 | 4006 Straight[A] or | | | | | | | standard patent |10.54| 11.99
```

|1.61| 75.36 |0.50| 0.09 | 4050 flour | | | | | | | First clear grade |10.13| 13.74
|2.20| 73.13 |0.80| 0.12 | 4097 flour | | | | | | | Second clear grade |10.08| 15.03
|3.77| 69.37 |1.75| 0.56 | 4267 flour | | | | | | | | "Red dog" flour | 9.17| 18.98
|7.00| 61.37 |3.48| 0.59 | 4485 Shorts | 8.73| 14.87 |6.37| 65.47 |4.56| 0.14 |
4414 Bran | 9.99| 14.02 |4.39| 65.54 |6.06| 0.23 | 4198 Entire-wheat flour
|10.81| 12.26 |2.24| 73.67 |1.02| 0.32 | 4032 Graham flour | 8.61| 12.65 |2.44|
74.58 |1.72| 0.18 | 4148 Wheat | 8.50| 12.65 |2.36| 74.69 |1.80| 0.18 | 4140

===

========================

[Footnote A: Straight flour includes the first and second patents and first clear grade.]

In the table it will be noted that there is a gradual increase in protein content from first patent to "red dog," the largest amount being in the "red dog" flour. Although "red dog" contains the most protein, it is by far the poorest flour in bread-making qualities, and in the milling of wheat often it is not separated from the offals, but is sold as an animal food. It will also be seen that there is a gradual increase in the ash content from the highest to the lowest grades of flour, the increase being practically proportional to the grade,--the most ash being in the lowest grade. The grade to which a flour belongs can be determined more accurately from the ash content than from any other constituent. Patent grades of flour rarely contain more than 0.55 per cent of ash,--the better grades less than 0.5 per cent. The more completely the bran and offals are removed during the process of milling, the lower the per cent of ash. The ash content, however, cannot be taken as an absolute guide in all cases, as noticeable variations occur in the amount of mineral matter or ash in different wheats; starchy wheats that have reached full maturity often contain less than hard wheats grown upon rich soil where the growing season has been short, and from such wheats a soft, straight flour may have as low a per cent of ash as a hard first patent flour. When only straight or standard patent flour is manufactured by a mill, all of the flour is included which would otherwise be designated first and second patents and first clear.

157. Graham and Entire Wheat Flours.--When the germ and a portion of the bran are retained in the flour, and the particles are not completely reduced, the product is called "entire wheat flour." The name does not accurately describe the product, as it includes all of the flour and only a portion of the bran, and not the entire wheat kernel. Graham flour is coarsely granulated wheat meal. No sieves or bolting cloths are employed in its manufacture, and many coarse, unpulverized particles are present in the product[62].

158. Composition of Wheat Offals.--Bran and shorts are characterized by a high percentage of fiber, or cellulose. The ash, fat, and protein content of bran are all larger than of flour. The protein, however, is not in the form of gluten, but is largely albumin and globulins,[16] which are mainly in the aleurone layer of the wheat kernel, and are inclosed in branny capsules, and consequently are in a form not readily digested by man.

The germ is generally included in the shorts, although occasionally it is removed for special commercial purposes. It is sometimes sterilized and used in breakfast food products. The germ is rich in oil and is excluded from the flour mainly because it has a tendency to become rancid and to impart to the flour poor keeping qualities. Wheat oil has cathartic properties, and it is believed the physiological action of whole wheat and graham bread is in part due to the oil. The germ is also rich in protein, mainly in the form of globulins and proteoses. A dough cannot be made of pure germ, because it contains so little of the gliadin and glutenin.

159. Aging and Curing of Flour.--Flours well milled and made from high-grade, cleaned wheat generally improve in bread-making value when stored in clean, ventilated warehouses for periods of three to six months[9]. High-grade flour becomes drier and whiter and produces bread of slightly better quality when properly cured by storage. If the flour is in any way unsound, it deteriorates during storage, due to the action of ferment bodies. Wheat also, when properly cleaned and stored, improves in milling and bread-making

value. Certain enzymic changes appear to take place which are beneficial. Wheats differ materially from year to year in bread-making value, and those produced in seasons when all the conditions for crop growth are normal do not seem to be so much improved by storing and aging, either of the wheat or the flour, as when the growing season has been unfavorable. When wheat is stored, specific changes occur in both the germ and the cells of the kernel; these changes are akin to the ripening process, and appear to be greater if, for any reason, the wheat has failed to fully mature or is abnormal in composition.

The flour yield of wheat is in general proportional to the weight per bushel of the grain, well-filled, heavy grain producing more flour than light grain.[61] The quality of the flour, however, is not necessarily proportional to the weight of the grain. It is often necessary to blend different grades and types of wheat in order to secure good flour.

160. Macaroni Flour is made from durum wheat, according to Saunders a variety of hard, spring wheat. It is best grown in regions of restricted rainfall. Durum and other varieties of hard spring wheat grown under similar conditions, differ but little in general chemical composition, except that the gluten of durum appears to have a different percentage of gliadin and glutenin, and the flour has a more decided yellow color. Durum wheats are not generally considered as valuable for bread making as other hard wheat. They differ widely in bread-making value, some being very poor, while others produce bread of fair quality.[68]

161. Color.--The highest grades of flour are white in color, or of a slight creamy tinge. Dark-colored, slaty, and gray flours are of inferior quality, indicating a poor grade of wheat, poor milling, or a poor quality of gluten. Flours, after being on the market for a time, bleach a little and improve to a slight degree in color. Color is one of the characteristics by which the commercial value of flour is determined; the whiter the flour, the better the grade, provided other properties are equal[9]. The color, however, should be a pure or cream white. Some flours have what is called a dead white color,

and, while not objectionable as far as color is concerned, they are not as valuable for bread-making and general commercial purposes. One of the principal trade requirements of a flour is that it possess a certain degree of whiteness and none of the objectionable shades mentioned.

To determine the color of a flour, it is compared with a standard. If it is a winter wheat flour, one of the best high-grade winter patents to be found on the market is selected, and the sample in question is compared with this; if it is a spring wheat patent flour, one of the best spring wheat patent grades is taken as the standard. In making the comparison, the flours should be placed side by side on a glass plate and smoothed with the flour trier, the comparison being made preferably by a north window. Much experience and practice are necessary in order to determine with accuracy the color value of a flour.

162. Granulation.--The best patent grades of flour contain an appreciable amount of granular middlings, which have a characteristic "feel" similar to fine, sharp sand. A flour which has no granular feeling is not usually considered of the highest grade, but is generally a soft wheat flour of poor gluten. However, a flour should not be too coarsely granulated. The percentage amounts of the different grades of stock in a flour can be approximately determined by means of sieves and different sized bolting cloths. To test a flour, ten grams are placed in a sieve containing a No. 10 bolting cloth; with a camel's-hair brush and proper manipulation, the flour is sieved, and that which passes through is weighed. The percentage amount remaining on the No. 10 cloth is coarser middlings. Nearly all high-grade flours leave no residue on the No. 10 cloth. The sifted flour from the No. 10 cloth is also passed through Nos. 11, 12, 13, and 14 cloths[63]. In this way the approximate granulation of any grade of flour may be determined, and the granulation of an unknown sample be compared with that of a standard flour. In determining the granulation of a flour, if there are any coarse or discolored particles of bran or dust, they should be noted, as it is an indication of poor milling. When the flour is smoothed with a trier, there should be no channels formed on the surface of the flour, due to fibrous

impurities caught under the edge of the trier. A hand magnifying glass is useful for detecting the presence of abnormal amounts of dirt or fibrous matter in the flour.

163. Capacity of Flour to absorb Water.--The capacity of a flour to absorb water is determined by adding water from a burette to a weighed amount of flour until a dough of standard consistency is obtained. Low absorption is due to low gluten content. A good flour should absorb from 60 to 65 per cent of its weight of water. In making the test, it is advisable to determine the absorption of a flour of known baking value at the same time that an unknown flour is being tested. Flours of low absorption do not make breads of the best quality; also there are a smaller number of loaves per barrel, and the bread dries out more readily.

164. Physical Properties of Gluten.--The percentages of wet and dry gluten in a flour are determined as outlined in Experiment No. 27. Flours of good character should show at least 30 per cent moist gluten and from 10 to 12 per cent dry gluten. The quality of a flour is not necessarily proportional to its gluten content, although a flour with less than 10-1/2 per cent of dry gluten will not make the best quality of bread, and flours with excessive amounts are sometimes poor bread makers. The color of the gluten is also important; it should be white or creamy. The statements made in regard to color of flour apply also to color of the gluten. A dark, stringy, or putty-like gluten is of little value for bread-making purposes.[64] In making the gluten test, it is advisable to compare the gluten with that from a flour of known bread-making value. Soft wheat flours have a gluten of different character from hard wheat flours.

165. Gluten as a Factor in Bread Making.--The bread-making value of a flour is dependent upon the character of the wheat and the method of milling. It is not necessarily dependent upon the amount of gluten, as the largest volume and best quality of bread are often made from flour of average rather than maximum gluten content. But flours with low gluten do not produce high-grade breads. When a flour contains more than 12 or 13 per cent of

proteids, any increase does not necessarily mean added bread-making value. The quality of the gluten, equally with the amount, determines the value for bread-making purposes.

166. Unsoundness.--A flour with more than 14 per cent of moisture is liable to become unsound. High acidity also is an indication of unsoundness or of poor keeping qualities. The odor of a sample of flour should always be carefully noted, for any suggestion of fermentation sufficient to affect the odor renders the flour unsuited for making the best bread. Any abnormal odor in flour is objectionable, as it is due to contamination of some sort, and most frequently to fermentation changes. A musty odor is always an indication of unsoundness. Some flours which have but a slight suggestion of mustiness will, when baked into bread, have it more pronounced; on the other hand, some odors are removed during bread making. Flours may absorb odors because of being stored in contaminated places or being shipped in cars in which oil or other ill-smelling products with strong odors have previously been shipped. Unsoundness is often due to faulty methods in handling, as well as to poor wheat, or to lack of proper cleaning of the wheat or flour.

167. Comparative Baking Tests.--To determine the bread-making value of a flour, comparative baking tests, as outlined in Experiment No. 29, are made; the flour in question is thus compared as to bread-making value with a flour of known baking quality. In making the baking tests, the absorption of the flour, the way in which it responds in the doughing process, and the general properties of the dough, are noted. The details should be carried out with care, the comparison always being made with a similar flour of known baking value, and the bread should be baked at the same time and under the same conditions as the standard. The color of the bread, the size and weight of the loaf, and its texture and odor, are the principal characteristics to be noted.

The quality of flour for bread-making purposes is not strictly dependent upon any one factor, but appears to be the aggregate of a number of desirable characteristics. The commercial grade of a flour can be accurately determined from the color, granulation, absorption, gluten and ash content, and the quality of the bread. Technical flour testing requires much experience and a high degree of skill.

168. Bleaching.--In the process of manufacture, flours are often subjected to air containing traces of nitrogen peroxide gas, generated by electrical action and resulting in the union of the oxygen and nitrogen of the air. This whitens and improves the color of the flour. Bleached flours differ neither in chemical composition nor in nutritive value from unbleached flours, except that bleached flours contain a small amount (about one part to one million parts of flour) of nitrite reacting material, which is removed during the process of bread making. The amount of nitrites produced in flour during bleaching is less than is normally present in the saliva, or is found naturally in many vegetable foods, or in smoked or cured meats, or in bread made from unbleached flour and baked in a gas oven where nitrites are produced from combustion of the gas. The bleaching of flour cannot be regarded as in any way injurious to health or as adulteration, and a bleached flour which has good gluten and bread-making qualities is entirely satisfactory. It is not possible to successfully bleach low-grade flours so they will resemble the high grades, because the bran impurities of the low grades blacken during bleaching and become more prominent. Alway, of the Nebraska Experiment Station, has shown that there is no danger to apprehend from over-bleaching, for when excess of the bleaching reagent is used, flours become yellow in color[65]. Similar results have been obtained at the Minnesota Experiment Station. As bleaching is not injurious to health, and as it is not possible through bleaching to change low grades so as to resemble the patent grades, bleaching resolves itself entirely into the question of what color of flour the consumer desires. Pending the settlement of the status of bleaching the practice has been largely discontinued.

169. Adulteration of Flour.--Flour is not easily adulterated, as the addition of any foreign material interferes with the expansion and bread-making qualities and hence is readily detected. The mixing of other cereals, as corn

flour, with wheat flour has been attempted at various times when wheat commanded a high price, but this also is readily detected, by microscopic examination, as the corn starch and wheat starch grains are quite different in mechanical structure. Such flours are required to be labeled, in accord with the congressional act of 1898, when Congress passed, in advance of the general pure food bill, an act regulating the labeling and sale of mixed and adulterated flours. Various statements have been made in regard to the adulteration of flour with minerals, as chalk and barytes, but such adulteration does not appear to be at all general.

170. Nutritive Value of Flour.--From a nutritive point of view, wheat flour and wheat bread have a high value.[66] A larger amount of nutrients can be secured for a given sum of money in the form of flour than of any other food material except corn meal. According to statistics, the average per capita consumption of wheat in the United States is about 4-1/2 bushels, or, approximately, one barrel per year, and from recent investigations it would appear that the amount of flour used in the dietary is on the increase. According to the Bureau of Labor, flour costs the average laborer about one tenth as much as all other foods combined, although he secures from it a proportionally larger amount of nutritive material than from any other food.

CHAPTER XI

BREAD AND BREAD MAKING

171. Leavened and Unleavened Bread.--To make unleavened bread the flour is moistened and worked into a stiff dough, which is then rolled thin, cut into various shapes, and baked, forming a brittle biscuit or cracker.

The process of making raised or leavened bread consists, in brief, of mixing the flour and water in proper proportions for a stiff dough, together with some salt for seasoning, and yeast (or other agent) for leavening. The moistened gluten of the flour forms a viscid, elastic, tenacious mass, which is thoroughly kneaded to distribute the yeast. The dough is then set in a warm place and the yeast begins to grow, or "work," causing alcoholic fermentation, with the production of carbon dioxid gas, which expands the dough, or causes it to "rise," thus rendering it porous. After the yeast has grown sufficiently, the dough is baked in a hot oven, where further fermentation is stopped because of destruction of the yeast by the heat, which also causes the gas to expand the loaf and, in addition, generates steam. The gas and steam inflate the tenacious dough and finally escape into the oven. At the same time the gluten of the dough is hardened by the heat, and the mass remains porous and light, while the outer surface is darkened and formed into a crust.

When the flour is of good quality, the dough well prepared, and the bread properly baked, the loaf has certain definite characteristics. It should be well raised and have a thin, flinty crust, which is not too dark in color nor too tough, but which cracks when broken; the crumb, as the interior of the loaf is called, should be porous, elastic, and of uniform texture, without large holes, and should have good flavor, odor, and color.

Meal or flour from any of the cereals may be used for unleavened bread, but leavened bread can be made only from those that contain gluten, a mixture of vegetable proteids which when moistened with water becomes viscid, and is tenacious enough to confine the gas produced in the dough. Most cereals, as barley, rice, oats, and corn, some of which are very frequently made into forms of unleavened bread, are deficient or wholly lacking in gluten, and hence cannot be used alone for making leavened bread. For the leavened bread, wheat and rye, which contain an abundance of gluten, are best fitted, wheat being in this country by far the more commonly used.

172. Changes during Bread Making.--In bread making complex physical, chemical, and biological changes occur. Each chemical compound of the flour undergoes some change during the process. The most important changes are as follows[64]:

1. Production of carbon dioxid gas, alcohol, and soluble carbohydrates as the result of ferment action.

2. Partial rupturing of the starch grains and formation of a small amount of soluble carbohydrates due to the action of heat.

3. Production of lactic and other organic acids.

4. Formation of volatile carbon compounds, other than alcohol and carbon dioxid.

5. Change in the solubility of the gluten proteins, due to the action of the organic acids and fermentation.

6. Changes in the solubility of the proteids due to the action of heat, as coagulation of the albumin and globulin.

7. Formation and liberation of a small amount of volatile, nitrogenous compounds, as ammonia and amids.

8. Partial oxidation of the fat.

173. Loss of Dry Matter during Bread Making.--As many of the compounds formed during bread making are gases resulting from fermentation action, and as these are volatile at the temperature of baking, appreciable losses necessarily take place. Experiments show about 2 per cent of loss of dry matter under ordinary conditions. These losses are not confined to the carbohydrates alone, but also extend to the proteids and other compounds. When 100 pounds of flour containing 10 per cent of water and 90 per cent of dry matter are made into bread, the bread contains about 88 pounds of dry matter. In exceptional cases, where there has been prolonged fermentation, the losses exceed 2 per cent[64].

174. Action of Yeast.--Yeast is a monocellular plant requiring sugar and

other food materials for its nourishment. Under favorable conditions it rapidly increases by budding, and as a result produces the well-known alcoholic fermentation. It requires mineral food, as do plants of a higher order, and oftentimes the fermentation process is checked for want of sufficient soluble mineral food. The yeast plant causes a number of chemical changes to take place, as conversion of starch to a soluble form and alcoholic fermentation.

$$C_6H_{10}O_5 + H_2O = C_6H_{12}O_6.$$

$$C_6H_{12}O_6 = 2 C_2H_5OH + 2 CO_2.$$

Alcoholic fermentation cannot occur until the starch has been converted into dextrose sugar. The yeast plant is destroyed at a temperature of 131?F. It is most active from 70?to 90?F. At a low temperature it is less active, and when it freezes the cells are ruptured. A number of different kinds of fermentation are associated with the growth of the yeast plant, and there are many varieties of yeast, some of which are more active than others. For bread making an active yeast is desirable to prevent the formation of acid bodies. If the work proceeds quickly, the rising process is completed before the acid fermentation is far advanced. If fermentation is too prolonged, some of the products of the yeast plant impart an undesirable taste and odor to the bread, and hinder the development of the gluten and expansion of the loaf.

175. Compressed Yeast.--The yeast most commonly used in bread making is compressed yeast, a product of distilleries. The yeast floating on the surface of the wort is skimmed off and that remaining is allowed to settle to the bottom, and is obtained by running the wort into shallow tanks or settling trays. It is then washed with cold water, and the impurities are removed either by sieving through silk or wire sieves, or, during the washing, by fractional precipitation. The yeast is then pressed, cut into cakes, and wrapped in tinfoil. When fresh, it is of uniform creamy color, moist, and of a firm, even texture[18]. It should be kept cold, as it readily decomposes.

176. Dry Yeast is made by mixing starch or meal with fresh yeast until a stiff dough is formed. This is then dried, either in the sun or at a moderate temperature, and cut into cakes. By drying, many of the yeast cells are rendered temporarily inactive, and so it is a slower acting leaven than the compressed yeast. A dry yeast will keep indefinitely.

177. Production of Carbon Dioxid Gas and Alcohol.--Carbon dioxid and alcohol are produced in the largest amounts of any of the compounds formed during bread making. When the alcoholic ferments secreted by the yeast plant act upon the invert sugars and produce alcoholic fermentation, carbon dioxid is one of the products formed. Ordinarily about 1 per cent of carbon dioxid gas is generated and lost during bread making. About equal weights of carbon dioxid and alcohol are produced during the fermentation. In baking, the alcohol is vaporized and aids the carbon dioxid in expanding the dough and making the bread porous. If all of the moisture given off during bread making be collected it will be found that from a pound loaf of bread there are about 40 cubic centimeters of liquid; when this is submitted to chemical analysis, small amounts of alcohol are obtained. Alcoholic fermentation sometimes fails to take place readily, because there are not sufficient soluble carbohydrates to undergo inversion, or other food for the yeast plant. Starch cannot be converted directly into alcohol and carbon dioxid gas; it must first be changed into dextrose sugars, and these undergo alcoholic fermentation. Bread gives no appreciable reaction for alcohol even when fresh.[64]

If the gluten is of poor quality, or deficient in either gliadin or glutenin, the dough mass fails to properly expand because the gas is not all retained. The amount of gas formed is dependent upon temperature, rapidity of the ferment action, and quality of the yeast and flour. If the yeast is inactive, other forms of fermentation than the alcoholic may take place and, as a result, the dough does not expand. Poor yeast is a frequent cause of poor bread.

The temperature reached in bread making is not sufficient to destroy all the ferment bodies associated with the yeast, as, for example, bread sometimes becomes soft and stringy, due to fermentation changes after the bread has been baked and stored. Both bread and flour are subject to many bacterial diseases, and one of the objects of thorough cleaning of the wheat and removal of the bran and debris particles during the process of flour manufacture is to completely eliminate all ferment bodies mechanically associated with the exterior of the wheat kernel, which, if retained in the flour, would cause it readily to become unsound.

178. Production of Soluble Carbohydrates.--Flour contains naturally a small amount of soluble carbohydrates, which are readily acted upon by the alcoholic ferments. The yeast plant secretes soluble ferments, which act upon the starch, forming soluble carbohydrates, and the heat during baking brings about similar changes. In fact, soluble carbohydrates are both consumed and produced by ferment action during the bread-making process. Flour contains, on an average, 65 per cent of starch, and during bread making about 10 per cent is changed to soluble forms. Bread, on a dry matter basis, contains approximately 6 per cent of soluble carbohydrates, including dextrine, dextrose, and sucrose sugars.[64]

The physical changes which the starch grains undergo are also noticeable. Wheat starch has the structure shown in illustration No. 33. The starch grains are circular bodies, concave, with slight markings in the form of concentric rings. When the proteid matter of bread is extracted with alcohol and the starch grains are examined, it will, be seen that some of them are partially ruptured, like those in popped corn, while others have been slightly acted upon or eaten away by the organized ferments, the surface of the starch grains being pitted, as shown in the illustration. The joint action of heat and ferments on the starch grains changes them physically so they may more readily undergo digestion. The brown coating or crust formed upon the surface of bread is mainly dextrine, produced by the action of heat on the starch. Dextrine is a soluble carbohydrate, having the same general composition as starch, but differing from it in physical properties and ease of digestion.

179. Production of Acids in Bread Making.--Wheat bread made with yeast gives an acid reaction. The acid is produced from the carbohydrates by ferment action. Flour contains about one tenth of 1 per cent of acid; the dough contains from 0.3 to 0.5 per cent, while the baked bread contains from 0.14 to 0.3 per cent, but after two or three days slightly more acid is developed.[64] During the process of bread making, a small portion of the acid is volatilized, but the larger part enters into chemical combination with the gliadin, forming an acid proteid. When the alcoholic fermentation of bread making becomes less active, acid fermentations begin, and sour dough results. It is not definitely known what specific organic acids are developed in bread making. Lactic and butyric acids are known to be formed, and for purposes of calculation, the total acidity is expressed in terms of lactic acid.

The acidity is determined by weighing 20 grams of flour into a flask, adding 200 cubic centimeters of distilled water, shaking vigorously, and leaving the flour in contact with the water for an hour; 50 cubic centimeters of the filtered solution are then titrated with a tenth normal solution of potassium hydroxid. Phenolphthalein is used as the indicator. It cannot be said that all of the alkali is used for neutralizing the acid, as a portion enters into chemical combination with the proteids. If the method for determining the acid be varied, constant results are not secured. Unsound or musty flours usually show a high per cent of acidity.

180. Volatile Compounds produced during Bread Making.--In addition to carbon dioxid and alcohol, there is lost during bread making a small amount of carbon in other forms, as volatile acids and hydrocarbon products equivalent to about one tenth of one per cent of carbon dioxid. The aroma of freshly baked bread is due to these compounds. Both the odor and flavor of bread are caused in part by the volatile acids and hydrocarbons. The amount and kind of volatile products formed can be somewhat regulated through the fermentation process by the use of special flours and the addition of materials that produce specific fermentation changes and desirable aromatic compounds. Some of the ferment bodies left in flour from the imperfect

removal of the dirt adhering to the exterior of the wheat kernels impart characteristic flavors to the bread. The so-called nutty flavor of some bread is due to the action of these ferment bodies and, when intensified, it becomes objectionable. Fungous growths in unsound flour and bread result in the liberation of volatile products, which impart a musty odor. Good odor and flavor are very desirable in both flour and bread.

181. Behavior of Wheat Proteids in Bread Making.--Gluten is an ingredient of the flour on which its bread-making properties largely depend. The important thing, however, is not entirely the quantity of gluten, but more particularly its character. Two flours containing the same amounts of carbohydrates and proteid compounds, when converted into bread by exactly the same process, may produce bread of entirely different physical characteristics because of differences in the nature of the gluten of the two samples. Gluten is composed of two bodies called gliadin and glutenin. The gliadin, a sort of plant gelatin, is the material which binds the flour particles together to form the dough, thus giving it tenacity and adhesiveness; and the glutenin is the material to which the gliadin adheres. If there is an excess of gliadin, the dough is soft and sticky, while if there is a deficiency, it lacks expansive power. Many flours containing a large amount of gluten and total proteid material and possessing a high nutritive value, do not yield bread of the best quality, because of an imperfect blending of the gliadin and glutenin. This question is of much importance in the milling of wheats, especially in the blending of the different types of wheat. An abnormally large amount of gluten does not yield a correspondingly large loaf.

Experiments were made at the Minnesota Experiment Station to determine the relation between the nature of the gluten and the character of the bread. This was done by comparing bread from normal flour with that from other flour of the same lot, but having part or all of its gliadin extracted.[64] Dough made from the latter was not sticky, but felt like putty, and broke in the same way. The yeast caused the mass to expand a little when first placed in the oven; then the loaf broke apart at the top and decreased in size. When baked it was less than half the size of that from the same weight of normal flour, and decidedly inferior in other respects. The removal of part of the gliadin produced nearly the same effect as the extraction of the whole of it, and even when an equal quantity of normal flour was mixed with that from which part of the gliadin had been extracted, the bread was only slightly improved. In flour of the highest bread-making properties the two constituents, gliadin and glutenin, are present in such proportions as to form a well-balanced gluten.

The proteids of wheat flour are mainly in an insoluble form, although there are small amounts of albumins and globulins; these are coagulated by the action of heat during the bread-making process, and rendered insoluble. A portion of the acid that is developed unites with the gliadin and glutenin, forming acid proteids, which change the physical properties of the dough. Both gliadin and glutenin take important parts in bread making. The removal of gliadin from flour causes complete loss of bread-making properties. Ordinarily from 45 to 65 per cent of the total nitrogen of the flour is present in alcohol soluble or gliadin form. Proteids also undergo hydration during mixing, some water being chemically united with them, changing their physical properties. This hydration change is necessary for the full development of the physical properties of the gluten. The water and salt soluble proteids appear to take no important part in the bread-making process, as their removal in no way affects the size of the loaf or general character of the bread. Because of the action of the acids upon the gliadin, bread contains a larger amount of alcohol soluble nitrogen or gliadin than the flour from which the bread was made. It is believed that this action changes the molecular structure of the protein so that it is more readily separated into its component parts when it undergoes digestion and assimilation.

182. Production of Volatile Nitrogenous Compounds.--When fermentation is unnecessarily prolonged, an appreciable amount of nitrogen is volatilized in the form of ammonia and allied bodies, as amids. During the process of bread making, the yeast appears to act upon the protein, as well as upon the carbohydrates, and, as previously stated, losses of dry matter fall alike upon

these two classes of compounds, nitrogenous and non-nitrogenous. Analyses of the flours and materials used in bread making, and of the bread, show that ordinarily about 1.5 per cent of the total nitrogen is liberated in the form of gas during the bread-making process, and analyses of the gases dispelled in baking show approximately the same per cent of nitrogen. When bread is dried, as in a drying oven, a small amount of volatile nitrogen appears to be given off,--probably as ammonium compounds formed during fermentation. The nitrogen lost in bread making under ordinary conditions is not sufficient to affect the nutritive value of the product. The losses of both nitrogen and carbon are more than offset by the increased solubility of the proteids and carbohydrates, the preliminary changes they have undergone making them more digestible and valuable for food purposes. The nitrogen volatilized in bread making appears to be mainly that present in the flour in amid forms or liberated as the result of fermentation processes. The more stable proteids undergo only limited changes in solubility and are not volatilized.

183. Oxidation of Fat.--Flour contains about 1.25 per cent of fat mechanically mixed with a small amount of yellow coloring matter. During the process of bread making the fat undergoes slight oxidation, accompanied by changes in both physical and chemical properties. The fat from bread, when no lard or shortening has been added, is darker in color, more viscous, less soluble in ether, and has a lower iodine number, than fat from flour. The change in solubility of the fat is not, however, such as to affect food value, because the fat is not volatilized, and is only changed by the addition of a small amount of oxygen from the air. When wheat fat and other vegetable and animal fats are exposed to the air, they undergo changes known as aging, similar to the slight oxidation changes in bread making.[64]

184. Influence of the Addition of Wheat Starch and Gluten to Flour.--Ten per cent or more of starch may be added to normal flour containing a well-balanced gluten, without decreasing the size of the loaf. When moist gluten was added to flour, thus increasing the total amount of gluten, the size of the loaf was not increased[67].

	SIZE OF LOAF	WEIGHT
Wheat flour, 14 ounces	22-1/2 ?17-1/2	18.75
Wheat flour, 10% wheat starch	23-1/2 ?17	18.25
Wheat flour, 12.2% wheat starch	21-1/2 ?17	18.00
Wheat flour, 210 grams, about 8 ounces	12-3/4 ?9	12.00
Wheat flour, 10% gluten added, 210 grams	12-1/2 ?9	12.75
Wheat flour, 20% gluten added	12 ?8-3/4	13.00

So long as the quality of the gluten is not destroyed, the addition of a small amount of either starch or gluten to flour does not affect the size of the loaf, but removal of the gluten affects the moisture content and physical properties of the bread. The addition of starch to flour has the same effect upon the bread as the use of low gluten flour,--lessening the capacity of the flour to absorb water and producing a dryer bread of poorer quality.

185. Composition of Bread.--The composition of bread depends primarily upon that of the flour from which it was made. If milk and butter (or lard) are used in making the dough, as is commonly the case, their nutrients are, of course, added to those of the flour; but when only water and flour are used, the nutrients of the bread are simply those of the flour. In either case the amount of nutrients in the bread is smaller than in the same weight of flour, because a considerable part of the water or milk used in making the dough is present in the bread after baking; that is, a pound of bread contains less of any of the nutrients than a pound of the flour from which the bread was made, because the proportion of water in the bread is greater. The following table shows how the composition of flour compares with that of bread, the different kinds of bread all having been made from the flour with which they are compared:

COMPOSITION OF FLOUR, AND BREAD MADE FROM IT IN DIFFERENT WAYS

MATERIAL	WATER	PROTEIN	FAT	C.H.	ASH
	%	%	%	%	%
Flour	10.11	12.47	0.86	76.09	0.47
Bread from flour and water	36.12	9.46	0.40	53.70	0.32
Bread from flour, water, and lard	37.70	9.27	1.02	51.70	0.31
Bread from flour and skim milk	36.02	10.57	0.48	52.63	0.30

Thus it may be seen that the proportion of water is larger and of each nutrient smaller in bread than in flour, and that the nutrients of the flour are increased by those in the materials added in making the bread.

It is apparent that two breads of the same lot of flour may differ, according to the method used in making, and also that two loaves of bread made by exactly the same process but from different lots of flour, even when of the same grade or brand, do not necessarily have the same composition, because of possible variation in the flours. In bread made from flour of low gluten content, the per cent of protein is correspondingly low.

186. Use of Skim Milk and Lard in Bread Making.--When flours low in gluten are used, skim milk may be employed advantageously in making the bread, to increase the protein content. Tests show that such bread contains about 1 per cent more protein than that made with water. Ordinarily there is no gain from a nutritive point of view in adding an excessive amount of lard or other shortening, as it tends to widen the nutritive ratio.

187. Influence of Warm and Cold Flours on Bread Making.--When flour is stored in a cold closet or storeroom, it is not in condition to produce a good

quality of bread until it has been warmed to a temperature of about 70?F. Cold flour checks the fermentation process, and is occasionally the cause of poor bread. On the other hand, when flour is too warm (98?F.) the influence upon fermentation is unfavorable. Heating of flour does not affect the bread-making value, provided the flour is not heated above 158?F. and is subsequently cooled to a temperature of 70?F. Wheat flour contains naturally a number of ferment substances, some of which are destroyed by the action of heat. The natural ferments, or enzymes, of flour appear to take a part in bread making, imparting characteristic odors and flavors to the product.

188. Variations in the Process of Bread Making.--Since flours differ so in chemical composition, and the yeast plant acts upon all the compounds of flour, it naturally follows that bread making is not a simple but a complex operation, resulting in a number of intricate chemical reactions, which it is necessary to control and many of which are only imperfectly understood. Bread of the best physical quality and commercial value is made of flour from fully matured, hard wheats, containing a low per cent of acid, no foreign ferment materials or their products, and at least 12-1/2 per cent of proteids, of which the larger portion is in the form of gliadin. It is believed that a better quality of bread could be produced from many flours by slight changes or modifications in the process of bread making. It cannot be expected that the same process will give the best results alike with all types and kinds of flour. The kind of fermentation process that will produce the best bread from a given type of flour can be determined only by experimentation. Poor bread making is due as often to lack of skill on the part of the bread maker, and to poor yeast, as it is to poor quality of flour. Frequently the flour is blamed when the poor bread is due to other factors. Lack of control of the fermentation process, and the consequent development of acid and other organisms which check the activity of the alcoholic ferments, is a frequent cause of poor bread.

189. Digestibility of Bread.--Extensive experiments have been made by the Office of Experiment Stations of the United States Department of

Agriculture, at the Minnesota and Maine Experiment Stations, to determine the digestibility and nutritive value of bread. Different kinds and types of wheat were milled so as to secure from each three flours: graham, entire wheat, and standard patent. The flours were made into bread, and the bread fed to workingmen, and its digestibility determined. The experiments taken as a whole show that bread is an exceedingly digestible food, nearly 98 per cent of the starch or carbohydrate nutrients and about 88 per cent of the gluten or proteid constituents being assimilated by the body. In the case of the graham and entire wheat flours, although they contained a larger total amount of protein, the nutrients were not as completely digested and absorbed by the body as were those of the white flour. The body secured a larger amount of nutrients from the white than from the other grades of flour, the digestibility of the three types being as follows: standard patent flour, protein 88.6 per cent and carbohydrates 97.7 per cent; entire wheat flour, protein 82 percent and carbohydrates 93.5 per cent; graham flour, protein 74.9 per cent and carbohydrates 89.2 per cent. The low digestibility of the protein of the graham and entire wheat flours is supposed to be due to the coarser granulation; the proteins, being embedded and surrounded with cellular tissue, escape the action of the digestive fluids. Microscopic examination of the feces showed that often entire starch grains were still inclosed in the woody coverings and consequently had failed to undergo digestion.[62], [64], [67], [86]

190. Use of Graham and Entire Wheat in the Dietary.--Entire wheat and graham flours should be included in the dietary of some persons, as they are often valuable because of their physiological action, the branny particles stimulating the process of digestion and encouraging peristaltic action. In the diet of the overfed, they are valuable for the smaller rather than the larger amount of nutrients they contain. Also they supply bulk and give the digestive tract needed exercise. For the laboring man, where it is necessary to obtain the largest amount of available nutrients, bread from white flour should be supplied; in the dietary of the sedentary, graham and entire wheat flours can, if found beneficial, be made to form an essential part. The kind of bread that it is best to use is largely a matter of personal choice founded

upon experience.

"When we pass on to consider the relative nutritive values of white and whole-meal bread, we are on ground that has been the scene of many a controversy. It is often contended that whole-meal is preferable to white bread, because it is richer in proteid and mineral matter, and so makes a better balanced diet. But our examination of the chemical composition of whole-meal bread has shown that as regards proteid at least, this is not always true, and even were it the case, the lesser absorption of whole-meal bread, which we have seen to occur, would tend to annul the advantage.... On the whole, we may fairly regard the vexed question of whole-meal versus white bread as finally settled and settled in favor of the latter."[28]

"The higher percentage of nitrogen in bran than in fine flour has frequently led to the recommendation of the coarser breads as more nutritious than the finer. We have already seen that the more branny portions of the grain also contain a much larger percentage of mineral matter. And, further, it is in the bran that the largest proportion of fatty matter--the non-nitrogenous substance of higher respiratory capacity which the wheat contains--is found. It is, however, we think, very questionable whether upon such data alone a valid opinion can be formed of the comparative values of bread made from the finer or courser flours ground from one and the same grain. Again, it is an indisputable fact that branny particles when admitted into the flour in the degree of imperfect division in which our ordinary milling processes leave them very considerably increase the peristaltic action, and hence the alimentary canal is cleared much more rapidly of its contents. It is also well known that the poorer classes almost invariably prefer the whiter bread, and among some of those who work the hardest and who consequently soonest appreciate a difference in nutritive quality (navvies, for example) it is distinctly stated that their preference for the whiter bread is founded on the fact that the browner passes through them too rapidly; consequently, before their systems have extracted from it as much nutritious matter as it ought to yield them.... In fact, all experience tends to show that the state as well as the chemical composition of our food must be considered; in other words, that the digestibility and aptitude for assimilation are not less important qualities than its ultimate composition.

"But to suppose that whole-wheat meal as ordinarily prepared is, as has generally been assumed, weight for weight more nutritious than ordinary bread flour is an utter fallacy founded on theoretical text-book dicta, not only entirely unsupported by experience, but inconsistent with it. In fact, it is just the poorer fed and the harder working that should have the ordinary flour bread rather than the whole-meal bread as hitherto prepared, and it is the overfed and the sedentary that should have such whole-meal bread. Lastly, if the whole grain were finely ground, it is by no means certain that the percentage of really nutritive nitrogenous matters would be higher than in ordinary bread flour, and it is quite a question whether the excess of earthy phosphates would not then be injurious."--LAWES AND GILBERT.[68]

* * * * *

"According to the chemical analysis of graham, entire wheat, and standard patent flours milled from the same lot of hard Scotch Fife spring wheat, the graham flour contained the highest and the patent flour the lowest percentage of total protein. But according to the results of digestion experiments with these flours the proportions of digestible or available protein and available energy in the patent flour were larger than in either the entire wheat or the graham flour. The lower digestibility of the protein of the latter is due to the fact that in both these flours a considerable portion of this constituent is contained in the coarser particles (bran), and so resists the action of the digestive juices and escapes digestion. Thus while there actually may be more protein in a given amount of graham or entire wheat flour than in the same weight of patent flour from the same wheat, the body obtains less of the protein and energy from the coarse flour than it does from the fine, because, although the including of the bran and germ increases the percentage of protein, it decreases its digestibility. By digestibility is meant the difference between the amounts of the several nutrients consumed and the amount excreted in the feces.

"The digestibility of first and second patent flours was not appreciably different from that of standard patent flour. The degree of digestibility of all these flours is high, due largely to their mechanical condition; that is, to the fact that they are finely ground."--SNYDER.[62]

For a more extended discussion of the subject, the student is referred to Bulletins 67, 101, and 126, Office of Experiment Stations, United States Department of Agriculture.

191. Mineral Content of White Bread.--Average flour contains from 0.4 to 0.5 of 1 per cent of ash or mineral matter, the larger portion being lime and magnesia and phosphate of potassium. It is argued by some that graham and entire wheat flours should be used liberally because of their larger mineral content and their greater richness in phosphates. In a mixed dietary, however, in which bread forms an essential part, there is always an excess of phosphates, and there is nothing to be gained by increasing the amount, as it only requires additional work of the kidneys for its removal. Few experiments have been made to determine the phosphorus requirements of the human body, but these indicate that it is unnecessary to increase the phosphate content of a mixed diet. It is estimated that less than two grams per day of phosphates are required to meet all of the needs of the body, and in an average mixed ration there are present from three to five grams and more. A large portion of the phosphate compounds of white bread is present in organic combinations, as lecithin and nucleated proteids, which are the most available forms, and more valuable for purposes of nutrition than the mineral phosphates. In the case of graham and entire wheat flours, a proportionally smaller amount of the phosphates are digested and assimilated than from the finer grades of flour.

192. Comparative Digestibility of New and Old Bread.--With healthy persons there is no difference whatever in the completeness of digestibility of old and new bread; one appears to be as thoroughly absorbed as the other.

In the case of some individuals with impaired digestion there may be a difference in the ease and comfort with which the two kinds of bread are digested, but this is due mainly to individuality and does not apply generally. The change which bread undergoes when it is kept for several days is largely a loss of moisture and development of a small amount of acid and other substances from the continued ferment action.

193. Different Kinds of Bread.--According to variations in method of preparation, there are different types and varieties of bread, as the "flat bread" of Scandinavian countries, unleavened bread, Vienna bread, salt rising bread, etc. Bread made with baking powder differs in no essential way from that made with yeast, except in the presence of the residue from the baking powder, discussed in Chapter XII. Biscuits, wheat cakes, crackers, and other food materials made principally from flour, have practically the same food value as bread. It makes but little difference in what way flour is prepared as food, for in its various forms it has practically the same digestibility and nutritive value.

194. Toast.--When bread is toasted there is no change in the percentage of total nutrients on a dry matter basis. The change is in solubility and form, and not in amount of nutrients available. Some of the starch becomes dextrine, which is more soluble and digestible.[5] Proteids, on the other hand, are rendered less soluble, which appears to slightly lower the digestion coefficient. They are somewhat more readily but not quite so completely digested as those of bread. Digestion experiments show that toast more readily yields to the diastase and other ferments than does wheat bread. Toasting brings about ease of digestion rather than increased completeness of the process. Toast is a sterile food, while bread often contains various ferments which have not been destroyed by baking. These undergo incubation during the process of digestion, particularly in the case of individuals with diseases of the digestive tract. With normal digestion, however, these ferment bodies do not develop to any appreciable extent, as the digestive tract disinfects itself. When the flour is prepared from well cleaned wheat and the ferment substances which are present mainly in the

bran particles have been removed, a flour of higher sanitary value is secured.

CHAPTER XII

BAKING POWDERS

195. General Composition.--All baking powders contain at least two materials; one of these has combined carbon dioxid in its composition, the other some acid constituent which serves to liberate the gas. The material from which the gas is obtained is almost invariably sodium bicarbonate, $NaHCO_3$, commonly known as "soda" or "saleratus." Ammonium carbonate has been used to some extent, but is very seldom used at the present time. The acid constituent may be one of several materials, the most common being cream of tartar, tartaric acid, calcium phosphate, or alum. These may be used separately or in combination. The various baking powders are designated according to the acid constituent, as "cream of tartar," "phosphate," and "alum" powders. All of them liberate carbon dioxid gas, but the products left in the food differ widely in nature and amount[69].

Baking powder is a chemical preparation which, when brought in contact with water, liberates carbon dioxid gas. The baking powder is mixed dry with flour, and when this is moistened the carbon dioxid that is liberated expands the dough. The action is similar to that of yeast except that in the case of yeast the gas is given off much more slowly and no residue is left in the bread. When baking powder is used, there is a residue left in the food which varies with the material in the powder. It is the nature and amount of this residue that is important and makes one baking powder more desirable than another.

196. Cream of Tartar Powders.--The acid ingredient of the cream of tartar powders is tartaric acid, $H_2C_4H_4O_6$. Cream of tartar is potassium acid tartrate, $KHC_4H_4O_6$; it contains one atom of replaceable hydrogen, which imparts the acid properties, and it is prepared from crude argol, a deposit of grape juice when wine is made. The residue from this

powder is sodium potassium tartrate, $NaKC_4H_4O_6$, commonly known as Rochelle salt. This is the active ingredient of Seidlitz powders and has a purgative effect when taken into the body. The dose as a purgative is from one half to one ounce. A loaf of bread as ordinarily made with cream of tartar powder contains about 160 grains of Rochelle salt, which is 45 grains more than is found in a Seidlitz powder, but the amount actually eaten at any one time is small and its physiological effect can probably be disregarded. When a cream of tartar baking powder is used, the reaction takes place according to the following equation:

$$188 \ 84 \ 210 \ 44 \ 18 \ HKH_4C_4O_6 + NaHCO_3 = KNaC_4H_4O_6$$
$$+ CO_2 + H_2O.$$

The crystallized Rochelle salt contains four molecules of water, so that, even allowing for some starch filler, there is very nearly as much weight of material (Rochelle salt) left in the food as there was of the original powder. If free tartaric acid were used instead of potassium acid tartrate, the reaction would be as follows:

$$150 \quad 168 \quad 230 \quad 88 \quad H_2C_4H_4O_6 \quad + \quad 2NaHCO_3 \quad =$$
$$Na_2C_2H_4O_6.2 \ H_2O + 2CO_2.$$

But the residue, sodium tartrate, is less in proportion. It has physiological properties very similar to Rochelle salt. Tartaric acid is seldom used alone, but very often in combination with cream of tartar. It is more expensive than cream of tartar; but not so much is required, and it is more rapid in action.

197. Phosphate Baking Powders.--Here the acid ingredient is phosphoric acid and the compound usually employed is mono-calcium phosphate, $CaH_4(PO-_4)_2$. This is made by the action of sulphuric acid on ground bone $(Ca_3(PO_4)_2 + 2 \ H_2SO_4 = CaH_4(PO_4)_2 + 2 \ CaSO_4)$, and it is difficult to free it from the calcium phosphate formed at the same time; hence such powders contain more or less of this inert material. The reaction which occurs with a phosphate powder is as follows:

$$234 \; 168 \; 136 \; CaH_4(PO_4)_2 + 2 \, NaHCO_3 = CaHPO_4$$

$$88 \; 36 \; 142 + 2 \, CO_2 + 2 \, H_2O + Na_2HPO_4.$$

Sodium phosphate, according to the United States Dispensatory, is "mildly purgative in doses of from 1 to 2 ounces." The claim is made by the makers of phosphate baking powders that the phosphates of sodium and calcium, products left after the baking, restore the phosphates which have been lost from the flour in the bran. This baking powder residue does not restore the phosphates in the same form in which they are present in grains and it does furnish them in larger amounts--nearly tenfold. However, the residue from these powders is probably less objectionable than that from alum powders. The chief drawback to the phosphate powders is their poor keeping qualities.

198. Alum Baking Powders.--Sulphuric acid is the acid constituent of these powders. The alums are double sulphates of aluminium and an alkali metal, and have the general formula $xAl(SO_4)_2$ in which x may be K, Na, or NH_4, producing respectively a potash, soda, or ammonia alum. Potash alum is most commonly used, soda and ammonia alums to a less extent. The reaction takes place as follows:

$$475 \; 504 \; 157 \; 2 \, NH_4Al(SO_4)_2 + 6 \, NaHCO_3 = Al_2(OH)_6$$

$$426 \; 132 \; 264 + 3 \, Na_2SO_4 + (NH_4)_2SO_4 + 6 \, CO_2.$$

If it is a potash or soda alum, simply substitute K or Na for NH_4 throughout the equation. The best authorities regard alum baking powders as the most objectionable. Ammonia alum is without doubt the worst form, since all of the ammonium compounds have an extremely irritating effect on animal tissue. Sulphates of sodium and potassium are also objectionable. Aluminium hydroxide is soluble in the slightly acid gastric juice and has an astringent action on animal tissue, hindering digestion in a way similar to the alum itself. Many of the alum powders contain also mono-calcium phosphate; the reaction is as follows:

$$475 \ 234 \ 336 \ \ 2\,NH_4Al(SO_4)_2 + CaH_4(PO_4)_2 + 4\,NaHCO_3$$

$$245 \ 136 \ 132 \ = Al_2(PO_4)_2 + CaSO_4 + (NH_4)_2SO_4$$

$$284 \ 176 \ 72 \ + 2\,Na_2SO_4 + 4\,CO_2 + 4\,H_2O.$$

These are probably less injurious than the straight alum powders, although the residues are, in general, open to the same objection.

199. Inspection of Baking Powders.--Many of the states have enacted laws seeking to regulate the sale of alum baking powders. Some of these laws simply require the packages to bear a label setting forth the fact that alum is one of the ingredients; others require the baking powder packages to bear a label naming all the ingredients of the powder.

200. Fillers.--All baking powders contain a filler of starch. This is necessary to keep the materials from acting before the powder is used. The amount of filler varies from 15 to 50 per cent; the least is found in the tartrate powders and the most in the phosphate powders. The amount of gas which a powder gives off regulates its value; it should give off at least 1/8 of its weight.

201. Home-made Baking Powders.--Baking powders can be made at home for about one half what they usually cost and they will give equal satisfaction. The following will make a long-keeping powder: cream of tartar, 8 ounces; baking soda, 4 ounces; corn starch, 3 ounces. For a quick-acting powder use but one ounce of starch. The materials should be thoroughly dry. Mix the soda and starch first by shaking well in a glass or tin can. Add the cream of tartar last and shake again. Thorough mixing is essential to good results. Cream of tartar is often adulterated, but it can be obtained pure from a reliable druggist. To insure baking powders remaining perfectly dry, they should always be kept in glass or tin cans, never in paper.

CHAPTER XIII

VINEGAR, SPICES, AND CONDIMENTS

202. Vinegar.--Vinegar is a dilute solution of acetic acid produced by fermentation, and contains, in addition to acetic acid, small amounts of other materials in solution, as mineral matter and malic acid, according to the material from which the vinegar was made. Unless otherwise designated, vinegar in this country is generally considered to be made from apples. Other substances, however, are used, as vinegar can be manufactured from a variety of fermentable materials, as molasses, glucose, malt, wine, and alcoholic beverages in general. The chemical changes which take place in the production of vinegars are: (1) inversion of the sugar, (2) conversion of the invert sugars into alcohol, and (3) change of alcohol into acetic acid. All these chemical changes are the result of ferment action. The various invert ferments change the sugar into dextrose and glucose sugars; then the alcoholic ferment produces alcohol and carbon dioxid from the invert sugars, and finally the acetic acid ferment completes the work by converting the alcohol into acetic acid. The chemical changes which take place in these different steps are:

sucrose dextrose levulose (1) $C_{12}H_{22}O_{11} + H_2O = C_6H_{12}O_6 + C_6H_{12}O_6$;

dextrose alcohol (2) $C_6H_{12}O_6 = 2\ C_2H_5OH + 2\ CO_2$;

alcohol acid (3) $C_2H_5OH + 2\ O = HC_2H_3O_2 + H_2O$.

The acetic acid organism, Mycoderma aceti, can work only in the presence of oxygen. It is one of the aerobic ferments, and is present in what is known as the "mother" of vinegar and is secreted by it. When vinegar is made in quantity, the process is hastened by allowing the alcoholic solution to pass through a narrow tank rilled with shavings containing some of the ferment material, and at the same time air is admitted so as to secure a good supply of oxygen. When vinegar is made by allowing cider or wine to stand in a warm place until the fermentation process is completed, a long time is required--the length of time depending upon the supply of air and other conditions affecting fermentation.

In some countries malt vinegar is common. This is produced by allowing a wort made from malt and barley to undergo acetic acid fermentation, without first distilling the alcohol as is done in the preparation of spirit vinegar. In various European countries wine vinegar is in general use and is made by acetification of the juice of grapes. Sometimes spirit vinegar is made from corn or barley malt. Alcoholic fermentation takes place, the alcohol is distilled so that a weak solution remains, which is acetified in the ordinary way. Such a vinegar can be produced very cheaply and is much inferior in flavor to genuine wine or cider vinegar.

Vinegar, when properly made, should remain clear, and should not form a heavy deposit or produce any large amount of the fungous growth, commonly called the "mother" of vinegar. In order to prevent the vinegar from becoming cloudy and forming deposits, it should be strained and stored in clean jugs and protected from the air. So long as air is excluded further acetic acid fermentation and production of "mother" of vinegar cannot take place. When the vinegar is properly made and the fermentation process has been completed, the acid already produced prevents all further development of acetic acid ferments. When vinegar becomes cloudy and produces deposits, it is an indication that the acetic fermentation has not been completed.

The national standard for pure apple cider vinegar calls for not less than 4 grams acetic acid, 1.6 grams of apple solids, and 0.25 grams of apple ash per 100 cubic centimeters, along with other characteristics, as acidity, sugar, and phosphoric acid content. Many states have special laws regarding the sale of vinegar.

203. Adulteration of Vinegar.--Vinegar is frequently adulterated by the addition of water, or by coloring spirit vinegar, thus causing it to resemble cider vinegar. Formerly vinegar was occasionally adulterated by the use of mineral acids, as hydrochloric or sulphuric, but since acetic acid can be produced so cheaply, this form of adulteration has almost entirely disappeared. Colored spirit vinegar contains merely a trace of solid matter and can be readily distinguished from cider vinegar by evaporating a small weighed quantity to dryness and determining the weight of the solids. Occasionally, however, glucose and other materials are added so as to give some solids to the spirit vinegar, but such a vinegar contains only a trace of ash[18]. Attempts have also been made to carry the adulteration still further by adding lime and soda to give the colored spirit vinegar the necessary amount of ash. Malt, white wine, glucose, and molasses vinegars when properly manufactured and unadulterated are not objectionable, but too frequently they are made to resemble and sell as cider vinegar. This is a fraud which affects the pocketbook rather than the health. For home use apple cider vinegar is highly desirable. There is no food material or food adjunct, unless possibly ground coffee and spices, so extensively adulterated as vinegar.

Vinegar has no food value whatever, and is valuable only for giving flavor and palatability to other foods, and to some extent for the preservation of foods. It is useful in the household in other ways, as it furnishes a dilute acid solution of aid in some cooking and baking operations for liberating gas from soda, and also when a dilute acid solution is required for various cleaning purposes.

Vinegar should never be kept in tin pails, or any metallic vessel, because the acetic acid readily dissolves copper, tin, iron, and the ordinary metals, producing poisonous solutions. Earthenware jugs, porcelain dishes, glassware, or wooden casks are all serviceable for storing vinegar.

204. Characteristics of Spices.[70]--Spices are aromatic vegetable substances characterized as a class by containing some essential or volatile

oil which gives taste and individuality to the material. They are used for the flavoring of food and are composed of mineral matter and the various nitrogenous and non-nitrogenous compounds found in all plant bodies. Since only a comparatively small amount of a spice is used for flavoring purposes, no appreciable nutrients are added to the food. Some of the spices have characteristic medicinal properties. Occasionally they are used to such an extent as to mask the natural flavors of foods, and to conceal poor cooking and preparation or poor quality. For the microscopic study of spices the student is referred to Winton, "Microscopy of Vegetable Foods," and Leach, "Food Inspection and Analysis."

205. Pepper.--Black and white pepper are the fruit of the pepper plant (Piper nigrum), a climbing perennial shrub which grows in the East and West Indies, the greatest production being in Sumatra. For the black pepper, the berry is picked before thoroughly ripe; for the white pepper, it is allowed to mature. White pepper has the black pericarp or hull removed. Pepper owes its properties to an alkaloid, piperine, and to a volatile oil. In the black pepper berries there is present ash to the extent of about 4.5 per cent, it ought not to be above 6.5 per cent; ether extract, including piperine and resin, not less than 6.5 per cent; crude fiber not more than 16 per cent; also some starch and nitrogenous material. The white pepper contains less ash and cellulose than the black pepper. Ground pepper is frequently grossly adulterated; common adulterants being: cracker crumbs, roasted nut shells and fruit stones, charcoal, corn meal, pepper hulls, mustard hulls, and buckwheat middlings. The pepper berries wrinkle in drying, and this makes it difficult to remove the sand which may have adhered to them. An excessive amount of sand in the ash should be classed as adulteration. Adulterants in pepper are detected mainly by the use of the microscope. The United States standard for pepper is: not more than 7 per cent total ash, 15 per cent fiber, and not less than 25 per cent starch and 6 per cent non-volatile ether extract.[71]

206. Cayenne.--Cayenne or red pepper is the fruit pod of a plant, capsicum, of which there are several varieties,--the small-fruited kind, used to make

cayenne or red pepper; and the tabasco sort, forming the basis of tabasco sauce. It is grown mainly in the tropics, and was used there as a condiment before the landing of Columbus, who took specimens back to Europe. Cayenne pepper contains 25 per cent of oil, about 7 per cent of ash, and a liberal amount of starch. The adulterants are usually of a starchy nature, as rice or corn meal, and the product is often colored with some red dye.

207. Mustard.--Mustard is the seed of the mustard plant, and is most often found in commerce in the ground form. The black or brown mustard has a very small seed and the most aroma. White mustard is much larger and is frequently used unground. For the ground mustard, only the interior of the seed is used, the husk being removed in the bolting. Mustard contains a large amount of oil, part of which is usually expressed before grinding, and this is the form in which spice grinders buy it. In mustard flour there is: ash from 4 to 6 per cent, volatile oil from 0.5 to 2 per cent, fixed oil from 15 to 25 per cent, crude fiber from 2 to 5 per cent, albuminoids from 35 to 45 per cent, and a little starch. The principal adulterants are wheat, corn, and rice flour. When these are used, the product is frequently colored with turmeric, a harmless vegetable coloring material.

208. Ginger.--Ginger is the rhizome or root of a reed-like plant (Zingiber officinale), native in tropical Asia, chiefly India. It is cultivated in nearly all tropical countries. When unground it usually occurs in two forms: dried with the epidermis, or with the epidermis removed, when it is called scraped ginger. Very frequently a coating of chalk is given, as a protection against the drug store beetle. Jamaica ginger is the best and most expensive. Cochin, scraped, African, and Calcutta ginger range in price in the order given. Ginger contains from 3.6 to 7.5 per cent of ash, from 1.5 to 3 per cent of volatile oil, and from 3 to 5.5 per cent of fixed oil. There is a large amount of starch. The chief adulterants are rice, wheat, and potato starch, mustard hulls, exhausted ginger from ginger-ale and extract factories, sawdust and ground peanut-shells, and turmeric is frequently used for coloring the product. The United States standard for ginger is not more than 42 per cent starch, 8 per cent fiber, and 6 per cent total ash.[71]

209. Cinnamon and Cassia.--The bark of several species of plants growing in tropical countries furnishes these spices. True cinnamon is a native of Ceylon, while the cassias are from Bengal and China. In this country there is more cassia used than cinnamon--cinnamon being rarely found except in drug stores. Cassia bark is much thicker than cinnamon bark. The ground spice contains about 1.5 per cent volatile oil and the same amount of fixed oil, 4 per cent of ash, and some fiber, nitrogenous matter, and starch. Cereals, cedar sawdust, ground nutshells, oil meal, and cracker crumbs are the chief adulterants.

210. Cloves.--Cloves are the flower buds of an evergreen tree that grows in the tropics. These are picked by hand and dried in the sun. In the order of value, Penang, Sumatra, Amboyna, and Zanzibar furnish the chief varieties. Cloves rarely contain more than 8 per cent ash, or less than 10 per cent volatile oil and 4 per cent fixed oil, and 16 to 20 per cent of tannin-yielding bodies. No starch is present. The chief adulterants of ground cloves are spent cloves, allspice, and ground nutshells. Clove stems are also sometimes used and may be detected by a microscopical examination, since they contain many thick-walled cells and much fibrous tissue.

211. Allspice.--Allspice, or pimento, is the fruit of an evergreen tree common in the West Indies. It is a small, dry, globular berry, two-celled, each cell having a single seed. Allspice contains about 2.5 per cent volatile oil, 4 per cent fixed oil, and 4.5 per cent ash. Because of its cheapness, it is not generally adulterated, cereal starches being the most common adulterants.

212. Nutmeg.--Nutmeg is the interior kernel of the fruit of a tree growing in the East Indies. The fruit resembles a small pear. A fleshy mantle of crimson color, which is mace, envelopes the seed. Nutmeg contains about 2.2 per cent ash, 2.5 to 5 per cent volatile oil, and 25 to 35 per cent fixed oil. Mace has practically the same composition. Extensive adulteration is seldom practiced. The white coating on the surface of the nutmeg is lime, used to prevent sprouting of the germ.

CHAPTER XIV

TEA, COFFEE, CHOCOLATE, AND COCOA

213. Tea is the prepared leaf of an evergreen shrub or small tree cultivated chiefly in China and Japan. There are two varieties of plants. The Assamese, which requires a very moist, hot climate, yields in India and Ceylon about 400 pounds per acre, and may produce as high as 1000 pounds. From this plant a number of flushes or pickings are secured in a year. The Chinese plant grows in cooler climates and has a smaller, tougher, and darker leaf, which is more delicate than that of the Assamese and is usually made into green tea. The Chinese tea plant yields only four or five flushes a year. About 40 per cent of the tea used in this country comes from Japan and 50 per cent from China. The tea industry of India and Ceylon has developed rapidly in late years, and is now second only to that of China. Tea has been raised upon a small scale in the United States. The quality or grade of the tea depends upon the leaves used and the method of curing.

214. Composition of Tea.--Black and green teas are produced from the same species of plant, but owe their difference in color as well as flavor and odor to methods of preparation. The same plant may yield several grades of both green and black tea. To produce black tea, the leaves are bruised to liberate the juices, allowed to ferment a short time, which develops the color, and then dried.[73] For green tea the fresh leaves are roasted or steamed, then rolled and dried as quickly as possible to prevent fermentation. The smaller leaves and the first picking produce the finest quality of tea. The characteristic flavor and odor of tea are imparted by a volatile oil, although the odor is sometimes altered by the tea being brought in contact with orange flowers, jessamine, or the fragrant olive. There are also present in tea an alkaloid, theine, which gives the peculiar physiological properties, and tannin, upon which depends largely the strength of the tea infusion. The composition of tea is as follows:

GREEN | BLACK | TEA | TEA | TEA

	GREEN TEA	BLACK TEA	TEA
Tannin, per cent	12.91	10.64	4.89
Theine, per cent	3.30	3.20	3.30
Ash, per cent	4.97	4.92	4.93
Fiber, per cent	10.44	10.06	10.07
Protein, per cent	37.33	37.43	38.90 (all insoluble)

It will be noticed that green tea contains twice as much tannin as black tea; during the fermentation which the black tea undergoes, some of the tannin is decomposed. There is a large amount of protein in tea, but it is of no food value, because of its insolubility. About half of the ash is soluble. The tannin is readily soluble, and for this reason green tea especially should be infused for a very short time and never boiled. Tannin in foods in large amounts may interfere with the normal digestion of the protein compounds, because it coagulates the albumin and peptones after they have become soluble, and thus makes additional work for the digestive organs.

215. Judging Teas.--Teas are judged according to: (1) the tea as it appears prepared for market, (2) the infusion, and (3) the out-turn after infusion. The color should be uniform; if a black tea, it should be grayish black, not a dead black. The leaves should be uniform in size or grade. The quality and grade are dependent upon flavor, and, with the strength of the infusion, are determined by tasting. This work is rapidly done by the trained tea taster. The out-turn should be of one color; no bright green leaves should be present; evenness of make is judged by the out-turn. The flavor of a tea is largely a matter of personal judgment, but from a physiological point of view black teas are given the preference.

216. Adulteration of Tea.--A few years ago tea was quite extensively adulterated, but the strict regulation of the government regarding imported tea has greatly lessened adulteration. The most common form was the use of spent leaves, i.e. leaves which had been infused. Leaves of the willow and other plants which resemble tea were also used, as well as large quantities of tea stems. Facing or coloring is also an adulteration, since it is done to give

poor or damaged tea a brighter appearance. "Facing consists in treating leaves damaged in manufacture or which from age are inferior, with a mixture containing Prussian blue, turmeric, indigo, or plumbago to impart color or gloss, and with a fraudulent intent. There is no evidence that the facing agents are deleterious to health in the small quantities used, but as they are used for purposes of deception, they should be discouraged."[73] Facing and the addition of stems are the chief adulterations practiced at present.

217. Food Value and Physiological Properties of Tea.--Tea infusion does not contain sufficient nutrients to entitle it to be classed as a food. It is with some persons a stimulant. The caffein or theine in tea is an alkaloid that has characteristic physiological properties. In doses of from three to five grains, according to the United States Dispensatory, "it produces peculiar wakefulness." Larger doses produce intense physical restlessness, mental anxiety, and obstinate sleeplessness. "It has no effect upon the motor nerves, but is believed to have a visible effect upon the sensatory nerves." (United States Dispensatory.) Experiments with animals show that it causes elevation of the arterial pressure. It is used as a cardiac stimulant. The quantity of theine consumed in a cup of tea is about 4/5 of a grain, or 1/4 of a medicinal dose.

1, Mocha; 2, Java; 3, Rio.]

218. Composition of Coffee.--The coffee tree is an evergreen cultivated in the tropics. It grows to a height of 30 feet, but when cultivated is kept pruned to from 6 to 10 feet. The fruit, which resembles a small cherry, with two seeds or coffee grains embedded in the pulp, is dried and the seeds removed, cleaned, and graded. Coffee has an entirely different composition from tea; it is characterized by a high per cent of fat and soluble carbohydrates, and also contains an essential oil and caffein, an alkaloid identical with theine. Tannic acid, not as free acid, is combined with caffein as a tannate.

COFFEE|ROASTED COFFEE ------------------------------------- | Per Cent |
Per Cent Water | 11.23 | 1.15 Ash | 3.92 | 4.75 Fat | 12.27 | 14.48 Sugar, etc. |
0.66 | 8.55 Protein | 12.07 | 13.98 Caffein | 1.21 | 1.24
===

The high per cent of sugar and other soluble carbohydrates in roasted coffee is caused by the action of heat upon the non-nitrogenous compounds. Coffee cannot be considered a food, because only a comparatively small amount of the nutrients are soluble and available. It is a mildly stimulating beverage. With some individuals it appears to promote the digestive process, while with others its effect is not beneficial. Coffee is more extensively used in this country than tea, and is subject to greater adulteration. It is adulterated by facing and glazing; i.e. coloring the berries to resemble different grades and coating them with caramel and dextrine. Spent coffee grains and coffee that has been extracted without grinding are also used as adulterants. Imitation berries made of rye, corn, or wheat paste, molded, colored with caramel, and baked have been found mixed with genuine coffee berries. Roasted cereals and chicory are used extensively to adulterate ground coffee. Chicory is prepared from the root of the chicory plant, which belongs to the same family as the dandelion. It is claimed by some that a small amount of chicory improves the flavor of coffee. However, when chicory is added to coffee, it should be so stated on the label and the amount used given. The dextrine and sugar used in glazing are browned or caramelized during roasting and impart a darker color to the infusion, making it appear better than it really is. The glazing also makes the coffee retain moisture which would otherwise be driven off during roasting. Coffee contains such a large per cent of oil that the berries generally float when thrown on water, while the imitation berries sink. Chicory also sinks rapidly and colors the water brown, while the coffee remains floating for some time.

There are three kinds of coffee in general use: Java, Mocha, and Rio or Brazil. The Brazil coffee has the largest berry and is usually styled by dealers as "low" or "low middlings." The Java coffee berries are smaller and paler in color, the better grades being brown. Mocha usually commands the highest price in commerce. The seeds are small and dark yellow before roasting.

219. Cereal Coffee Substitutes.

"A few of these preparations contain a little true coffee, but for the most part they appear to be made of parched grains of barley, wheat, etc., or of grain mixed with pea hulls, ground corncobs, or wheat middlings. It is said that barley or wheat parched, with a little molasses, in an ordinary oven, makes something indistinguishable in flavor from some of the cereal coffees on the market. If no coffee is used in the cereal preparations, the claim that they are not stimulating is probably true. As for the nutritive value, parching the cereals undoubtedly renders some of the carbohydrates soluble, and a part of this soluble matter passes into the decoction, but the nutritive value of the infusion is hardly worth considering in the dietary."[56]

220. Cocoa and Chocolate Preparations.--Cocoa and chocolate are manufactured from the "cocoa bean," the seed of a tree native to tropical America. The beans are inclosed in a lemon-yellow, fleshy pod. They are removed from the pulp, allowed to undergo fermentation, and dried by exposure to the air and light, which hardens them and gives them a red color. This method produces what is known as the "fermented cocoa." For the "unfermented cocoa," the beans are dried without undergoing fermentation. Fermentation removes much of the acidity and bitterness characteristic to the unfermented bean, and when properly regulated develops flavor. The original bean contains about 50 per cent fat, part of which is removed in preparing the cocoa. This fat is sold as cocoa butter. In the preparation of some brands of cocoa, alkalies, such as soda and potash, are used to form a combination with the fat to prevent its separating in oily globules. This treatment improves the appearance of the cocoa, but experiments show the albumin to be somewhat less digestible and the soap-like product resulting not as valuable a food as the fat. Such preparations have a high per cent of ash. There is no objection from a nutritive point of view to a cocoa in which the fat separates in oily globules.

221. Composition of Cocoa.--The cocoa bean, when dried or roasted and freed from its husk and ground, is sold as cracked cocoa, or cocoa nibs. From cocoa nibs the various cocoa and chocolate preparations are made. Cocoas vary in composition according to the extent to which the fat is removed during the process of manufacture and the nature and extent to which other ingredients are added. An average cocoa contains about 20 per cent of proteids, and 30 per cent fat, also starch, sugar, gums, fiber, and ash, as well as theobromine, a material very similar to theine and caffein in tea and coffee, but not such an active stimulant. Cocoa is not easily soluble, but it may be ground so fine that a long time is required for its sedimentation; or sugar or other soluble material may be added during the process of manufacture to increase the specific gravity of the liquid to such an extent that the same object is attained without such fine grinding. The first method is to be preferred. Cocoa and its preparations are richer in nutritive substances than tea and coffee and have this added advantage that both the soluble and insoluble portions become a part of the beverage. Owing to the small amount used for a cup of cocoa, independent of the milk it does not add much in the way of nutrients to the ration.

222. Chocolate.--Plain chocolate is prepared from cocoa nibs without "removal of the fat or other constituents except the germ." It differs in chemical composition from cocoa by containing more fat and less protein; it has nearly the same chemical composition as the cocoa nibs. It is officially defined as containing "not more than 3 per cent of ash insoluble in water, 3-1/2 per cent of crude fiber and 9 per cent of starch, and less than 45 per cent cocoa fat."[71]

By the addition of sugar, sweet chocolates are made. They vary widely in composition according to the flavors and amounts of sugar added during their preparation. The average composition of cocoa nibs, standard cocoa, and plain chocolate is as follows:

	COCOA STANDARD COCOA	COMPOSITION OF PLAIN CHOCOLATE	COMPOSITION OF NIBS
	Per Cent	Per Cent	Per Cent
Water	3.00	--	3.09
Ash	3.50	4.20	3.08
Theobromine	1.00	--	--
Caffein	0.50	--	--
Crude Protein	12.00	--	--
Crude fiber	2.50	5.02	2.63
Fat	50.00	32.52	49.81
Starch and other non-nitrogenous matter	27.50	--	--

223. Adulteration of Chocolate and Cocoa.--The various chocolate and cocoa preparations offer an enticing field for sophistication; they are not, however, so extensively adulterated as before the enforcement of national and state pure food laws. The most common adulterants are starch, cocoa shells, and occasionally iron dioxid and other pigments to give color, also foreign fats to replace the fat removed and to give the required plasticity for molding.

224. Comparative Composition of Beverages.--Tea and coffee as beverages contain but little in the way of nutrients other than the cream and sugar used in them. The solid matter in tea and coffee infusions amounts to less than 1.2 per cent. When cocoa is made with milk, it is a beverage of high nutritive value due mainly to the milk.

COMPOSITION OF BEVERAGES[56]

KIND OF BEVERAGE PER LB.	WATER Per Cent	PROTEIN Per Cent	FAT Per Cent	CARBO-HYDRATES Per Cent	FUEL VALUE Calories
Commercial cereal coffee (0.5 ounce to 1 pint water)	98.2	0.2	--	1.4	30
Parched corn coffee (1.6 ounces to 1 pint water)	99.5	0.2	--	0.5	13
Oatmeal					

water (1 ounce | | | | | to 1 pint water) | 99.7 | 0.3 | -- | 0.3 | 11 Coffee (1 ounce | | | | | 1 pint water) | 98.9 | 0.2 | -- | 0.7 | 16 Tea (0.5 ounce to | | | | | 1 pint water) | 99.5 | 0.2 | -- | 0.6 | 15 Cocoa (0.5 ounce to | | | | | 1 pint milk) | 84.5 | 3.8 | 4.7 | 6.0 | 365 Cocoa (0.5 ounce to | | | | | 1 pint water) | 97.1 | 0.6 | 0.9 | 1.1 | 65 Skimmed milk | 90.5 | 3.4 | 0.3 | 5.1 | 170

===

===============================

CHAPTER XV

THE DIGESTIBILITY OF FOODS

225. Digestibility, How Determined.--The term "digestibility," as applied to foods, is used in two ways: (1) meaning the thoroughness of the process, or the completeness with which the nutrients of the food are absorbed and used by the body, and (2) meaning the ease or comfort with which digestion is accomplished. Cheese is popularly termed indigestible, and rice digestible, when in reality the nutrients of cheese are more completely although more slowly digested than those of rice. In this work, unless otherwise stated, digestibility is applied to the completeness of the digestion process.

The digestibility of a food is ascertained by means of digestion experiments, in which all of the food consumed for a certain period, usually two to four days, is weighed and analyzed, and from the weight and composition is determined the amount, in pounds or grams, of each nutrient consumed.[72] In like manner the nutrients in the indigestible portion, or feces, are determined from the weight and composition of the feces. The indigestible nutrients in the feces are deducted from the total nutrients of the food, the difference being the amount digested, or oxidized in the body. When the food is digested, the various nutrients undergo complete or partial oxidation, with the formation of carbon dioxid gas, water, urea (CH_4N_2O), and other compounds. The feces consist mainly of the compounds which have escaped digestion. The various groups of compounds of foods do not all have the same digestibility; for example, the starch of potatoes is 92 per cent digestible, while the protein is only 72 per cent. The percentage amount of a nutrient that is digested is called the digestion coefficient.

In the following way the digestibility of a two-days ration of bread and milk was determined: 773.5 grams of bread and 2000 grams of milk were consumed by the subject. The dried feces weighed 38.2 grams. The foods and feces when analyzed were found to have the following composition:[62]

COMPOSITION	BREAD	MILK	FECES[A]
Water	44.13	86.52	--
Crude protein	7.75	3.15	25.88
Ether extract	0.90	4.63	18.23
Ash	0.32	0.70	26.35
Carbohydrates	46.90	5.00	29.54
Calories per gram	2.450	0.79	5.083

[Footnote A: Results on dry-matter basis.]

STATEMENT OF RESULTS OF A DIGESTION EXPERIMENT

FOOD CONSUMED MATERIAL	WEIGHT	PROTEIN N ?6.25	ETHER EXTRACT	CARBO-HYDRATES	ASH	HEAT OF COMBUSTION
	Grams	Grams	Grams	Grams	Grams	Calories
Bread	773.5	60.0	6.9	362.8	2.5	1895
Milk	2000.0	63.0	92.6	100.0	14.0	1585
Total	38.2	123.0	99.5	462.8	16.5	3480
Feces		9.9	7.0	11.3	10.1	194
Total amount digested		113.1	92.5	451.5	6.4	3286
Per cent digested or coefficients of digestibility		92.0	93.0	97.5	38.8	94.4

| Available | energy | | | -- | | -- | | -- | | -- | | 90.0 |

==

=================================

In this experiment 92 per cent of the crude protein, 93 per cent of the ether extract, and 97.5 per cent of the carbohydrates of the bread and milk ration were digested and absorbed by the body. In calculating the available energy, correction is made for the unoxidized residue, as urea and allied forms. It is estimated that for each gram of protein in the ration there was an indigestible residue yielding 1.25 calories.

226. Available Nutrients.--A food may contain a comparatively large amount of a compound, and yet, on account of its low digestibility, fail to supply much of it to the body in an available form. Hence it is that the value of a food is dependent not alone on its composition, but also on its digestibility. The digestible or available nutrients of a food are determined by multiplying the per cent of each nutrient which the food contains by its digestion coefficient. For example, a sample of wheat flour contains 12 per cent protein, 88 per cent of which is digestible, making 10.56 per cent of available or digestible protein (12 ?0.88-10.56). Graham flour made from similar wheat contains 13 per cent total protein, and only 75 per cent of the protein is digestible, making 9.75 per cent available (13 ?0.75 = 9.75). Thus one food may contain a larger total but a smaller available amount of a nutrient than another.

227. Available Energy.--The available energy of a food or a ration is expressed in calories. A ration for a laborer at active out-of-door work should yield about 3200 calories. The calory is the unit of heat, and represents the heat required to raise the temperature of a kilogram of water 1?C., or four pounds of water 1?F. The caloric value of foods is determined by the calorimeter, an apparatus which measures heat with great accuracy. A pound of starch, or allied carbohydrates, yields 1860 calories, and a pound of fat 4225 (see Section 13). While a gram of protein completely burned produces 7.8 calories, digested it yields only about 4.2 calories, because, as

explained in the preceding section, not all of the carbon and oxygen are oxidized.[59] The caloric value or available energy of a ration can be calculated from the digestible nutrients by multiplying the pounds of digestible protein and carbohydrates by 1860, the digestible fat by 4225, and adding the results. For determination of the available energy of foods under different experimental conditions, and where great accuracy is desired, a specially constructed respiration calorimeter has been devised, which is built upon the same principle as an ordinary calorimeter, except it is large enough to admit a person, and is provided with appliances for measuring and analyzing the intake and outlet of air.[74] The heat produced by the combustion of the food in the body warms the water surrounding the calorimeter chamber, and this increase in temperature is determined by thermometers reading to 0.005 of a degree or less.

228. Normal Digestion and Health.--While the process of digestion has been extensively studied, it is not perfectly understood. Between the initial compounds of foods and their final oxidation products a large number of intermediate substances are formed, and when digestion fails to take place in a normal way, toxic or poisonous compounds are produced and various diseases result. It is probable that more diseases are due to imperfect or malnutrition than to any other cause. There is a very close relationship between health and normal digestion of the food.

The cells in the different parts of the digestive tract secrete fluids containing substances known as soluble ferments, or enzymes, which act upon the various compounds of foods, changing them chemically and physically so that they can be absorbed and utilized by the body. (See Section 31.) Some of the more important ferments are: ptyolin of the saliva, pepsin of the stomach, and pancreatin and diastase of the intestines. In order that these ferments may carry on their work in a normal way, the acidity and alkalinity of the different parts of the digestive tract must be maintained. The gastric juice contains from 0.1 to 0.25 per cent of hydrochloric acid, imparting mildly antiseptic properties; and while the peptic ferment works in a slightly acid solution, the tryptic ferment requires an alkaline solution. To secrete the necessary amount and quality of digestive fluids, the organs must be in a healthy condition. Many erroneous ideas regarding the digestion of foods are based upon misinterpretation of facts by persons suffering from impaired digestion, and attempts are frequently made to apply to normal digestion generalizations applicable only to diseased conditions.

229. Digestibility of Animal Foods.--The proteids and fats in animal foods, as meats, are more completely digested than the same class of nutrients in vegetables. In general, about 95 per cent of the proteids of meats is digestible, while those in vegetables are often less than 85 percent digestible. The amount of indigestible residue from animal foods is small; while from vegetables it is large, for the cellulose prevents complete absorption of the nutrients and, as a result, there is much indigestible residue. Animal foods are concentrated, in that they furnish large amounts of nutrients in digestible forms. There is less difference in the completeness with which various meats are digested than in their ease of digestion; the proteins all have about the same digestion coefficients, but vary with individuals as to ease of digestion and time required. It is generally considered that the digestible proteins, whether of animal or vegetable origin, are equally valuable for food purposes. This is an assumption, however, that has not been well established by experimental evidence. In a mixed ration, the proteins from different sources appear to have the same nutritive value, but as each is composed of different radicals and separated into dissimilar elementary compounds during the process of digestion, they would not necessarily all have the same food value.

There is but little difference between the fats and proteins of meats as to completeness of digestion,--the slight difference being in favor of the proteins. Some physiologists claim that the fat, which in some meats surrounds the bundles of fiber (protein), forming a protecting coat, prevents the complete solvent action of the digestive fluid. Very fat meats are not as completely digested as those moderately fat. It is also claimed that the digestibility of the meat is influenced by the mechanical character, as toughness of the fiber.

230. Digestibility of Vegetable Foods.--Vegetable foods vary in digestibility with their mechanical condition and the amount of cellulose or fiber. In some the nutrients are so embedded in cellular tissue as to be protected from the solvent action of the digestive fluids, and in such cases the digestibility and availability are low. The starches and sugars are more completely digested than any other of the nutrients of vegetables; in some instances they are from 95 to 98 per cent digestible. Some cellular tissue, but not an excess, is desirable in a ration, as it exerts a favorable mechanical action upon the organs of digestion, encourages peristalsis, and is an absorbent and dilutant of the waste products formed during digestion. For example, in the feeding of swine, it has been found that corn and cob meal often gives better results than corn fed alone. The cob contains but little in the way of nutrients, but it exerts a favorable mechanical action upon digestion. Occasionally too many bulky foods are combined, containing scant amounts of nutrients, so that the body receives insufficient protein. This is liable to be the case in the dietary of the strict vegetarian. Many of the vegetables possess special dietetic value, due to the organic acids and essential oils, as cited in the chapter on fruits and vegetables. The value of such foods cannot always be determined from their content of digestible protein, fat, and carbohydrates. This is particularly evident when they are omitted from the ration, as in the case of a restricted diet consisting mainly of animal foods. Many vegetables have low nutritive value on account of their bulky nature and the large amount of water and cellulose which they contain, which tends to decrease digestibility and lower the amount of available nutrients. Because of their bulk and fermentable nature, resulting in the formation of gases, a diet of coarse vegetables has a tendency to cause distention and enlargement of the intestinal organs. The carbohydrates, which are the chief constituents of vegetables, are digested mainly in the intestines, and require special mechanical preparation in the stomach, hence the nutrients of vegetables are not, as a rule, as easily digested as those of animal foods.

231. Factors influencing Digestion.--There are a number of factors which

influence completeness as well as ease of digestion, as: (1) combination of foods; (2) amount of food; (3) method of preparation; (4) mechanical condition of the food; (5) palatability; (6) physiological properties; (7) individuality of the consumer; and (8) psychological influences.

232. Combination of Foods.--In a mixed ration the nutrients are generally more completely digested than when only one food is used. For example, milk is practically all digested when it forms a part of a ration, and it also promotes digestibility of the foods with which it is combined, but when used alone it is less digestible.[27] Bread alone and milk alone are not as completely digested as bread and milk combined. The same in a general way has been observed in the feeding of farm animals,--better results are secured from combining two or more foods than from the use of one alone. The extent to which one food influences the digestibility of another has not been extensively studied.

In a mixed ration, consisting of several articles of food of different mechanical structure, the work of digestion is more evenly distributed among the various organs. A food often requires special preparation on the part of the stomach before it can be digested in the intestines, and if this food is consumed in small amounts and combined with others of different structure, the work of gastric digestion is lessened so that the foods are properly prepared and normal digestion takes place. The effect which one food exerts upon the digestibility of another is largely mechanical.

233. Amount of Food.--Completeness as well as ease of digestion is influenced by the amount of food consumed. In general, excessive amounts are not as completely digested as moderate amounts. In digestion experiments with oatmeal and milk, it was found that when these foods were consumed in large quantities the fat and protein were not as completely absorbed by the body as when less was used, the protein being 7 per cent and the fat 6 per cent more digestible in the medium ration. Experiments with animals show that economical results are not secured from an excess of food.[5] Some individuals consume too much food, and with them a

restricted diet would be beneficial, while others err in not consuming enough to meet the requirements of the body. Quite frequently it is those who need more food who practice dieting. When there is trouble with digestion, it is not always the amount or kind of food which is at fault, but other habits may be such as to affect digestion. The active out-of-door laborer can with impunity consume more food, because there is greater demand for nutrients, and the food is more completely oxidized in the body and without the formation of poisonous waste products. The amount of food consumed should be sufficient to meet all the demands of the body and maintain a normal weight.

234. Method of Preparation of Food.--The extent to which methods of cooking and preparation influence completeness of digestion has not been extensively investigated. As is well known, they have great influence upon ease and comfort of digestion. During cooking, as discussed in extensive physical and chemical changes occur, and these in turn affect digestibility. When the cooking has not been sufficient to mechanically disintegrate vegetable tissue, the digestive fluids fail to act favorably upon the food. Cooking is also beneficial because it renders the food sterile and destroys all objectionable microoganisms which, if they remain in food, readily undergo incubation in the digestive tract, interfering with normal digestion. Prolonged heat causes some foods to become less digestible, as milk, which digestion experiments show to be more completely digested when fresh than when sterilized. Pasteurized milk, which is not subjected to so high a temperature as sterilized milk, is more completely digested. See Chapter VII for discussion of sterilizing and pasteurizing milk.[38] The benefits derived from the destruction of the objectionable bacteria in foods are, however, greater than the losses attendant on lessened digestibility due to the action of heat. The method of preparation of a food affects its digestibility mainly through change in mechanical structure, and modification of the forms in which the nutrients are present.[5]

235. Mechanical Condition of Foods.--The mechanical condition of foods as to density and structure of the particles and the extent to which they are

disintegrated in their preparation for the table influences digestibility to a great extent. The mechanics of digestion is a subject that has not been extensively investigated, and it is one of great importance, as biological and chemical changes cannot take place if the food is not in proper mechanical condition. In general, the finer the food particles, the more completely the nutrients are acted upon by the digestive fluids and absorbed by the body. Nevertheless, the diet should not consist entirely of finely granulated foods. Some foods are valuable mainly because of the favorable action they exert mechanically upon digestion, rather than for the nutrients they contain.[62] Coarsely granulated breakfast foods, whole wheat flour, and many vegetables contain sufficient cellular tissue to give special value from a mechanical rather than a chemical point of view. The extent to which coarsely and finely granulated foods should enter into the ration is a question largely for the individual to determine. Experiments with pigs show that if large amounts of coarse, granular foods are consumed, the tendency is for the digestive tract to become inflamed and less able to exercise its normal functions. Coarsely granulated foods have a tendency to pass through the digestive tract in less time than those that are finely granulated, due largely to increased peristaltic action, and the result is the food is not retained a sufficient length of time to allow normal absorption to take place. In the feeding of farm animals, it has been found that the mechanical condition of the food has a great influence upon its economic use. Rations that are either too bulky or too concentrated fail to give the best results. In the human ration, the mechanical condition of the food is equally as important as its chemical composition.

236. Mastication is an important part of digestion, and when foods are not thoroughly masticated, additional work is required of the stomach, which is usually an overworked organ because of doing the work of the mouth as well. Although much of the mechanical preparation and mixing of foods is of necessity done in the stomach, some of it may advantageously be done in the mouth. The stomach should not be required to perform the function of the gizzard of a fowl.

237. Palatability of Foods.--Many foods naturally contain essential oils and other substances which impart palatability. These have but little in the way of nutritive value, but they assist in rendering the nutrients with which they are associated more digestible. Palatability of a food favorably influences the secretion of the gastric and other digestive fluids, and in this way the natural flavors of well-prepared foods aid in digestion. In the feeding of farm animals it has been found that when foods are consumed with a relish better returns are secured than when unpalatable foods are fed. To secure palatability the excessive use of condiments is unnecessary. It is possible to a great extent during preparation to develop and conserve the natural flavors. Some foods contain bitter principles which are removed during the cooking, while in others pleasant flavors are developed. Palatability is an important factor in the digestibility of foods.

238. Physiological Properties of Food.--Some food materials, particularly fruits and vegetables, contain compounds which have definite physiological properties, as tannin which is an astringent, special oils which exert a cathartic action, and the alkaloids which serve as irritants to nerve centers. Wheat germ oil is laxative, and it is probable that the physiological properties of graham and whole wheat breads are due in some degree to the oil which they contain.[67] The use of fruits, herbs, and vegetables for medicinal purposes is based upon the presence of compounds possessing well-defined medicinal properties. As a rule food plants do not contain appreciable amounts of such substances, and the use of food for medicinal effect should be by the advice of a physician. The physiological properties of some foods are due to bacterial products. See Chapter XX.

239. Individuality.--Material difference in digestive power is noticeable among individuals. Digestion experiments show that one person may digest 5 per cent more of a nutrient than another. This difference appears to be due to a number of factors, as activity of the organs, as affected by exercise and kind of labor performed; abnormal composition of the digestive fluids; or failure of the different parts of the digestive tract to act in harmony. Individuality is one of the most important factors in digestion. Persons

become accustomed to certain foods through long usage, and the digestive tract adapts itself to those foods, rendering sudden and extreme changes in the dietary hazardous. Common food articles may fail to properly digest in the case of some individuals, while with others they are consumed with benefit. What is food to one may prove to be a poison to another, and while general statements can be made in regard to the digestibility of foods, individual differences must be recognized.

240. Psychological Factors.--Previously conceived ideas concerning foods influence digestibility. Foods must be consumed with a relish in order to secure the best results, as flow of the digestive fluids and activity of the organs are to a certain extent dependent upon the nerve centers. If it is believed that a food is poisonous or injurious, even when the food is wholesome, normal digestion fails to take place. In experiments by the author, in which the comparative digestibility of butter and oleomargarine was being studied, it was found that when the subjects were told they were eating oleomargarine, its digestibility was depressed 5 per cent, and when they were not told the nature of the material, but assumed that butter was oleomargarine, the digestibility of the butter was lowered about 6 per cent.[13] Preconceived notions in regard to foods, not founded upon well-established facts, but due to prejudice resulting from ignorance, cause many valuable foods to be excluded from the dietary. Many persons, like the foreign lady who, visiting this country, said she ate only acquaintances, prefer foods that have a familiar taste and appearance, and any unusual taste or appearance detracts from the value because of the psychological influence upon digestion.

CHAPTER XVI

COMPARATIVE COST AND VALUE OF FOODS

241. Cost and Nutrient Content of Foods.--The market price and the nutritive value of foods are often at variance, as those which cost the most frequently contain the least nutrients.[75] It is difficult to make absolute

comparisons as to the nutritive value of foods at different prices, because they differ not only in the amounts, but also in the kinds of nutrients. While it is not possible to express definitely the value of one food in terms of another, approximate comparisons may be made as to the amounts of nutrients that can be secured for a given sum of money when foods are at different prices, and tables have been prepared making such comparisons.

242. Nutrients Procurable for a Given Sum.[7]--To ascertain the nutrients procurable for a given sum first determine the amount in pounds that can be obtained, say, for ten cents, and then multiply by the percentages of fat, protein, carbohydrates, and calories in the food. The results are the amounts, in pounds, of nutrients procurable for that sum of money. For example: if milk is 5 cents per quart, two quarts or approximately four pounds, can be procured for 10 cents. If the milk contains fat, 4 per cent, protein, 3.3 per cent, carbohydrates, 5 per cent, and fuel value, 310 calories per pound, multiplying each of these by 4 gives the nutrients and fuel value in four pounds, or 10 cents worth of milk, as follows:

Protein 0.13 lb. Fat 0.16 lb. Carbohydrates 0.2 lb. Calories 1240

If it is desired to compare milk at 5 cents per quart with round steak at 15 cents per pound, 10 cents will procure 0.66, or two thirds of a pound of round steak containing on an average (edible portion) 19 per cent protein, 12.8 per cent fat, and yielding 890 calories per pound. If 10 per cent is refuse, there is edible about 0.6 of a pound. The amounts of nutrients in the 0.6 of a pound of steak, edible portion, or 0.66 lb. as purchased would be:

Protein 0.11 lb. Fat 0.08 lb. Calories 534

It is to be observed that from the 10 cents' worth of milk a little more protein, 0.08 of a pound more fat, and nearly two and one half times as many calories can be secured as from the 10 cents' worth of meat. This is due to the carbohydrates and the larger amount of fat which the milk contains. At these prices, milk should be used liberally in the dietary, as it furnishes more of all the nutrients than does meat. It would not be advisable to exclude meat entirely from the ration, but milk at 5 cents per quart is cheaper food than meat at 15 cents per pound. In making comparisons, preference cannot always be given to one food because of its containing more of any particular nutrient, for often there are other factors that influence the value.

243. Comparing Foods as to Nutritive Value.--In general, preference should be given to foods which supply the most protein, provided the differences between the carbohydrates and fats are not large. When the protein content of two foods is nearly the same, but the fats and carbohydrates differ materially, the preference may safely be given to the food which supplies the larger amount of total nutrients. A pound of protein in a ration is more valuable than a pound of either fat or carbohydrates, although it is not possible to establish an absolute scale as to the comparative value of these nutrients, because they serve different functional purposes in the body. It is sometimes necessary to use small amounts of foods rich in protein in order to secure a balanced ration; excessive use of protein, however, is not economical, as that which is not needed for functional purposes is converted into heat and energy which could be supplied as well by the carbohydrates, and they are less expensive nutrients.

(From Office of Experiment Stations Bulletin.)]

TEN CENTS WILL PURCHASE: (From Farmer's Bulletin No. 142, U. S. Dept. of Agr.)

```
===================================================================
========================= | | TOTAL | | | | | | WEIGHT | | | | KIND OF
FOOD | PRICE | OF FOOD | | | CAR- | MATERIAL | PER | MATE-
|PROTEIN | FAT | BOHY- | ENERGY | POUND | RIAL | | | DRATES | -----
--------------------+-------+---------+--------+-------+---------+-------  | Cents |
Pounds | Pound | Pound | Pounds |Calories Beef, sirloin | 25 | 0.40 | 0.06 |
0.06 | -- | 410 Do. | 20 | 0.50 | 0.08 | 0.08 | -- | 515 Do. | 15 | 0.67 | 0.10 | 0.11
```

| -- | 685 Beef, round | 16 | 0.63 | 0.11 | 0.08 | -- | 560 Do. | 14 | 0.71 | 0.13 | 0.09 | -- | 630 Do. | 12 | 0.83 | 0.15 | 0.10 | -- | 740 Beef, shoulder clod | 12 | 0.83 | 0.13 | 0.08 | -- | 595 Do. | 9 | 1.11 | 0.18 | 0.10 | -- | 795 Beef, stew meat | 5 | 2.00 | 0.29 | 0.23 | -- | 1530 Beef, dried, chipped | 25 | 0.40 | 0.10 | 0.03 | -- | 315 Mutton chops, loin | 16 | 0.63 | 0.08 | 0.17 | -- | 890 Mutton, leg | 20 | 0.50 | 0.07 | 0.07 | -- | 445 Do. | 16 | 0.63 | 0.09 | 0.09 | -- | 560 Roast pork, loin | 12 | 0.83 | 0.11 | 0.19 | -- | 1035 Pork, smoked ham | 22 | 0.45 | 0.06 | 0.14 | -- | 735 Do. | 18 | 0.56 | 0.08 | 0.18 | -- | 915 Pork, fat salt | 12 | 0.83 | 0.02 | 0.68 | -- | 2950 Codfish, dressed, fresh | 10 | 1.00 | 0.11 | -- | -- | 220 Halibut, fresh | 18 | 0.56 | 0.08 | 0.02 | -- | 265 Cod, salt | 7 | 1.43 | 0.22 | 0.01 | -- | 465 Mackerel, salt, dressed | 10 | 1.00 | 0.13 | 0.20 | -- | 1135 Salmon, canned | 12 | 0.83 | 0.18 | 0.10 | -- | 760 Oysters, solids, | | | | | | 50 cents per quart | 25 | 0.40 | 0.02 | -- | 0.01 | 90 35 cents per quart | 18 | 0.56 | 0.03 | 0.01 | 0.02 | 125 Lobster, canned | 18 | 0.56 | 0.10 | 0.01 | -- | 225 Butter | 20 | 0.50 | 0.01 | 0.40 | -- | 1705 Do. | 25 | 0.40 | -- | 0.32 | -- | 1365 Do. | 30 | 0.33 | -- | 0.27 | -- | 1125 Eggs, 36 cents per dozen| 24 | 0.42 | 0.05 | 0.04 | -- | 260 Eggs, 24 cents per dozen| 16 | 0.63 | 0.07 | 0.06 | -- | 385 Eggs, 12 cents per dozen| 8 | 1.25 | 0.14 | 0.11 | -- | 770 Cheese | 16 | 0.63 | 0.16 | 0.20 | 0.02 | 1185 Milk, 7 cents per quart | 3-1/2 | 2.85 | 0.09 | 0.11 | 0.14 | 885 Milk, 6 cents per quart | 3 | 3.33 | 0.11 | 0.13 | 0.17 | 1030 Wheat flour | 3 | 3.33 | 0.32 | 0.03 | 2.45 | 5440 Do. | 2-1/2 | 4.00 | 0.39 | 0.04 | 2.94 | 6540 Corn meal, granular | 2-1/2 | 4.00 | 0.31 | 0.07 | 2.96 | 6540 Wheat breakfast food | 7-1/2 | 1.33 | 0.13 | 0.02 | 0.98 | 2235 Oat breakfast food | 7-1/2 | 1.33 | 0.19 | 0.09 | 0.86 | 2395 Oatmeal | 4 | 2.50 | 0.34 | 0.16 | 1.66 | 4500 Rice | 8 | 1.25 | 0.08 | -- | 0.97 | 2025 Wheat bread | 6 | 1.67 | 0.13 | 0.02 | 0.87 | 2000 Do. | 5 | 2.00 | 0.16 | 0.02 | 1.04 | 2400 Do. | 4 | 2.50 | 0.20 | 0.03 | 1.30 | 3000 Rye bread | 5 | 2.00 | 0.15 | 0.01 | 1.04 | 2340 Beans, white, dried | 5 | 2.00 | 0.35 | 0.03 | 1.16 | 3040 Cabbage | 2-1/2 | 4.00 | 0.05 | 0.01 | 0.18 | 460 Celery | 5 | 2.00 | 0.02 | -- | 0.05 | 130 Corn, canned | 10 | 1.00 | 0.02 | 0.01 | 0.18 | 430 Potatoes, | | | | | | 90 cents per bushel | 1-1/2| 6.67 | 0.10 | 0.01 | 0.93 | 1970 60 cents per bushel | 1 | 10.00 | 0.15 | 0.01 | 1.40 | 2950 45 cents per bushel | 3/4 | 13.33 | 0.20 | 0.01 | 1.87 | 3935 Turnips | 1 | 10.00 | 0.08 | 0.01 | 0.54 | 1200 Apples | 1-1/2| 6.67 | 0.02 | 0.02 | 0.65 | 1270 Bananas | 7 | 1.43 | 0.01 | 0.01 | 0.18 | 370 Oranges | 6 | 1.67 | 0.01 | -- | 0.13 | 250 Strawberries | 7 | 1.43 | .01 | 0.01

| 0.09 | 215 Sugar | 6 | 1.67 | -- | -- | 1.67 | 2920

==
==============================

It is to be noted in the table that, ordinarily, for the same amount of money the most nutrients can be obtained in the form of milk, cheese, sugar, and beans, corn meal, wheat flour, oatmeal, and cereals in bulk. While meats supply protein liberally, they fail to furnish carbohydrates as the vegetables. As discussed in the chapter on Dietary Studies of Families, unnecessarily expensive foods are often used, resulting either in lack of nutrients or unbalanced rations.

EXAMPLES

1. Compute the calories and the amounts of protein, fat, and carbohydrates that can be procured for 25 cents in cheese selling for 18 cents per pound; how do these compare with the nutrients in eggs at 20 cents per dozen?

2. Which food furnishes the larger amount of nutrients, potatoes at 50 cents per bushel or flour at $6 per barrel?

3. How do beans at 10 cents per quart compare in nutritive value with beef at 15 Cents per pound?

4. How does salt codfish at 10 cents per pound compare in nutritive value with lamb chops at 15 cents per pound?

5. Compare in nutritive value cream at 25 cents per quart with butter at 30 cents per pound.

6. Calculate the composition and nutritive value of a cake made of sugar, 8 oz.; butter, 4 oz.; eggs, 8 oz.; flour, 8 oz.; and milk, 4 oz.; the baked cake weighs one and three fourths pounds.

AVERAGE COMPOSITION OF COMMON AMERICAN FOOD PRODUCTS

(From Farmer's Bulletin, No. 142, U. S. Dept. of Agr.)

==
======================== | | | | | | | F | | | | | h | | up | R | | P | | C y | | e e |
e | W | r | | a d | | | l r | f | a | o | F | r r | A | Food Material | u | t | t | a | b a | s | v P
(as purchased) | s | e | e | t | o t | h | a o | e | r | i | | - e | | l u | | | n | | s | | u n | | | | |
| | e d -------------------------------+------+------+------+------+-----+-----+------ | |
| | | | | Calo- ANIMAL FOOD | % | % | % | % | % | % | ries | | | | | | | Beef, fresh:
| | | | | | | | Chuck ribs | 16.3 | 52.6 | 15.5 | 15.0 | -- | 0.8 | 910 Flank | 10.2 | 54.0 |
17.0 | 19.0 | -- | 0.7 | 1105 Loin | 13.3 | 52.5 | 16.1 | 17.5 | -- | 0.9 | 1025
Porterhouse steak | 12.7 | 52.4 | 19.1 | 17.9 | -- | 0.8 | 1100 Sirloin steak | 12.8
| 54.0 | 16.5 | 16.1 | -- | 0.9 | 975 Neck | 27.6 | 45.9 | 14.5 | 11.9 | -- | 0.7 | 1165
Ribs | 20.8 | 43.8 | 13.9 | 21.2 | -- | 0.7 | 1135 Rib rolls | -- | 63.9 | 19.3 | 16.7 |
-- | 0.9 | 1055 Round | 7.2 | 60.7 | 19.0 | 12.8 | -- | 1.0 | 890 Rump | 20.7 | 45.0
| 13.8 | 20.2 | -- | 0.7 | 1090 Shank, fore | 36.9 | 42.9 | 12.8 | 7.3 | -- | 0.6 | 545
Shoulder and clod | 16.4 | 56.8 | 16.4 | 9.8 | -- | 0.9 | 715 Fore quarter | 18.7 |
49.1 | 14.5 | 17.5 | -- | 0.7 | 995 Hind quarter | 15.7 | 50.4 | 15.4 | 18.3 | -- | 0.7
| 1045 Beef, corned, canned, | | | | | | | | pickled, dried: | | | | | | | | Corned beef | 8.4
| 49.2 | 14.3 | 23.8 | -- | 4.6 | 1245 Tongue, pickled | 6.0 | 58.9 | 11.9 | 19.2 | --
| 4.3 | 1010 Dried, salted, and smoked | 4.7 | 53.7 | 26.4 | 6.9 | -- | 8.9 | 790
Canned boiled beef | -- | 51.8 | 25.5 | 22.5 | -- | 1.3 | 1410 Canned corned beef
| -- | 51.8 | 26.3 | 18.7 | -- | 4.0 | 1270 Veal: | | | | | | | | Breast | 21.3 | 52.0 | 15.4 |
11.0 | -- | 0.8 | 745 Leg | 14.2 | 60.1 | 15.5 | 7.9 | -- | 0.9 | 625 Leg cutlets | 3.4
| 68.3 | 20.1 | 7.5 | -- | 1.0 | 695 Fore quarter | 24.5 | 54.2 | 15.1 | 6.0 | -- | 0.7 |
535 Hind quarter | 20.7 | 56.2 | 16.2 | 6.6 | -- | 0.8 | 580 Mutton: | | | | | | | | Flank
| 9.9 | 39.0 | 13.8 | 36.9 | -- | 0.6 | 1770 Leg, hind | 18.4 | 51.2 | 15.1 | 14.7 | -- |
0.8 | 890 Loin chops | 16.0 | 42.0 | 13.5 | 28.3 | -- | 0.7 | 1415 Fore quarter |
21.2 | 41.6 | 12.3 | 24.5 | -- | 0.7 | 1235 Hind quarter, without | 17.2 | 45.4 |
13.8 | 23.2 | -- | 0.7 | 1210 tallow | | | | | | | | Lamb: | | | | | | | | Breast | 10.1 | 45.5 |
15.4 | 19.1 | -- | 0.8 | 1075 Leg, hind | 17.4 | 52.9 | 15.9 | 13.6 | -- | 0.9 | 860

Pork, fresh: | | | | | | | Ham | 10.7 | 48.0 | 13.5 | 25.9 | -- | 0.8 | 1320 Loin chops | 19.7 | 41.8 | 13.4 | 24.2 | -- | 0.8 | 1245 Shoulder | 12.4 | 44.9 | 12.0 | 29.8 | -- | 0.7 | 1450 Tenderloin | -- | 66.5 | 18.9 | 13.0 | -- | 1.0 | 895 Pork, salted, cured, pickled: | | | | | | | Ham, smoked | 13.6 | 34.8 | 14.2 | 33.4 | -- | 4.2 | 1635 Shoulder, smoked | 18.2 | 36.8 | 13.0 | 26.6 | -- | 5.5 | 1335 Salt pork | -- | 7.9 | 1.9 | 86.2 | -- | 3.9 | 3555 Bacon, smoked | 7.7 | 17.4 | 9.1 | 62.2 | -- | 4.1 | 2715 Sausage: | | | | | | | Bologna | 3.3 | 55.2 | 18.2 | 19.7 | -- | 3.8 | 1155 Pork | -- | 39.8 | 13.0 | 44.2 | 1.1| 2.2 | 2075 Frankfort | -- | 57.2 | 19.6 | 18.6 | 1.1| 3.4 | 1155 Soups: | | | | | | | | Celery, cream of | -- | 88.6 | 2.1 | 2.8 | 5.0| 1.5 | 235 Beef | -- | 92.9 | 4.4 | 0.4 | 1.1| 1.2 | 120 Meat stew | -- | 84.5 | 4.6 | 4.3 | 5.5| 1.1 | 365 Tomato | -- | 90.0 | 1.8 | 1.1 | 5.6| 1.5 | 185 Poultry: | | | | | | | Chicken, broilers | 41.6 | 43.7 | 12.8 | 1.4 | -- | 0.7 | 305 Fowls | 25.9 | 47.1 | 13.7 | 12.3 | -- | 0.7 | 765 Goose | 17.6 | 38.5 | 13.4 | 29.8 | -- | 0.7 | 1475 Turkey | 22.7 | 42.4 | 16.1 | 18.4 | -- | 0.8 | 1060 Fish: | | | | | | | Cod, dressed | 29.9 | 58.5 | 11.1 | 0.2 | -- | 0.8 | 220 Halibut, steaks or sections | 17.7 | 61.9 | 15.3 | 4.4 | -- | 0.9 | 475 Mackerel, whole | 44.7 | 40.4 | 10.2 | 4.2 | -- | 0.7 | 370 Perch, yellow dressed | 35.1 | 50.7 | 12.8 | 0.7 | -- | 0.9 | 275 Shad, whole | 50.1 | 35.2 | 9.4 | 4.8 | -- | 0.7 | 380 Shad, roe | -- | 71.2 | 20.9 | 3.8 | 2.6| 1.5 | 600 Fish, preserved: | | | | | | | Cod, salt | 24.9 | 40.2 | 16.0 | 0.4 | -- |18.5 | 325 Herring, smoked | 44.4 | 19.2 | 20.5 | 8.8 | -- | 7.4 | 755 Fish, canned | | | | | | | Salmon | -- | 63.5 | 21.8 | 12.1 | -- | 2.6 | 915 Sardines |[A]5.0| 53.6 | 23.7 | 12.1 | -- | 5.3 | 950 Shellfish: | | | | | | | Clams | -- | 80.8 | 10.6 | 1.1 | 5.2 | 2.3| 340 Crabs | 52.4 | 36.7 | 7.9 | 0.9 | 0.6 | 1.5| 200 Lobsters | 61.7 | 30.7 | 5.9 | 0.7 | 0.2 | 0.8| 145 Eggs: Hen's eggs [B]|11.2 | 65.5 | 13.1 | 9.3 | -- | 0.9| 635 Dairy products, etc.: | | | | | | | Butter | -- | 11.0 | 1.0 |85.0 | -- | 3.0| 3410 Whole milk | -- | 87.0 | 3.3 | 4.0 | 5.0 | 0.7| 310 Skim milk | -- | 90.5 | 3.4 | 0.3 | 5.1 | 0.7| 165 Buttermilk | -- | 91.0 | 3.0 | 0.5 | 4.8 | 0.7| 160 Condensed milk | -- | 26.9 | 8.8 | 8.3 |54.1 | 1.9| 1430 Cream | -- | 74.0 | 2.5 |18.5 | 4.5 | 0.5| 865 Cheese, Cheddar | -- | 27.4 | 27.7 |36.8 | 4.1 | 4.0| 2075 Cheese, full cream | -- | 34.2 | 25.9 |33.7 | 2.4 | 3.8| 1885 | | | | | | | VEGETABLE FOOD | | | | | | | | | | | | | Flour, meal, etc.: | | | | | | | Entire wheat flour | -- | 11.4 | 13.8 | 1.9 |71.9 | 1.0| 1650 Graham flour | -- | 11.3 | 13.3 | 2.2 |71.4 | 1.8| 1645 Wheat flour, patent | | | | | | | roller process | | | | | | | High-grade and medium | -- | 12.0 | 11.4 | 1.0 |75.1 | 0.5| 1635 Low grade | -- | 12.0 | 14.0 | 1.9 |71.2 | 0.9| 1640 Macaroni, vermicelli, etc | -- | 10.3 | 13.4 | 0.9 |74.1 | 1.3| 1645 Wheat breakfast food | -- | 9.6 | 12.1 | 1.8 |75.2 | 1.3| 1680 Buckwheat flour | -- | 13.6 | 6.4 | 1.2 |77.9 | 0.9| 1605 Rye flour | -- | 12.9 | 6.8 | 0.9 |78.7 | 0.7| 1620 Corn meal | -- | 12.5 | 9.2 | 1.9 |75.4 | 1.0| 1635 Oat breakfast food | -- | 7.7 | 16.7 | 7.3 |66.2 | 2.1| 1800 Rice | -- | 12.3 | 8.0 | 0.3 |79.0 | 0.4| 1620 Tapioca | -- | 11.4 | 0.4 | 0.1 |88.0 | 0.1| 1650 Starch | -- | -- | -- | -- |90.0 | -- | 1675 Bread, pastry, etc.: | | | | | | | White bread | -- | 35.3 | 9.2 | 1.3 |53.1 | 1.1| 1200 Brown bread | -- | 43.6 | 5.4 | 1.8 |47.1 | 2.1| 1040 Bread, pastry, etc.: | | | | | | | | Graham bread | -- | 35.7 | 8.9 | 1.8| 52.1| 1.5 | 1195 Whole wheat bread | -- | 38.4 | 9.7.| 0.9| 49.7| 1.3 | 1130 Rye bread | -- | 35.7 | 9.0.| 0.6| 53.2| 1.5 | 1170 Cake | -- | 19.9 | 6.3.| 9.0| 63.3| 1.5 | 1630 Cream crackers | -- | 6.8 | 9.7.| 12.1| 69.7| 1.7 | 1925 Oyster crackers | -- | 4.8 | 11.3.| 10.5| 70.5| 2.9 | 1910 Soda crackers | -- | 5.9 | 9.8.| 9.1| 73.1| 2.1 | 1875 | | | | | | | Sugars, etc.: | | | | | | | | | | | | | | | | Molasses | -- | -- | -- | -- | 70.0| -- | 1225 Candy[C] | -- | -- | -- | -- | 96.0| -- | 1680 Honey | -- | -- | -- | -- | 81.0| -- | 1420 Sugar, granulated | -- | -- | -- | -- |100.0| -- | 1750 Maple sirup | -- | -- | -- | -- | 71.4| -- | 1250 | | | | | | | Vegetables:[D] | | | | | | | Beans, dried | -- | 12.6 | 22.5.| 1.8| 59.6| 3.5 | 1520 Beans, Lima, shelled | -- | 68.5 | 7.1.| 0.7| 22.0| 1.7 | 540 Beans, string | 7.0 | 83.0 | 2.1.| 0.3| 6.9| 0.7 | 170 Beets | 20.0 | 70.0 | 1.3.| 0.1| 7.7| 0.9 | 160 Cabbage | 15.0 | 77.7 | 1.4.| 0.2| 4.8| 0.9 | 115 Celery | 20.0 | 75.6 | 0.9.| 0.1| 2.6| 0.8 | 65 Corn, green (sweet), | | | | | | | edible portion | -- | 75.4 | 3.1 | 1.1| 19.7| 0.7 | 440 Cucumbers | 15.0 | 81.1 | 0.7.| 0.2| 2.6| 0.4 | 65 Lettuce | 15.0 | 80.5 | 1.0.| 0.2| 2.5| 0.8 | 65 Mushrooms | -- | 88.1 | 3.5 | 0.4| 6.8| 1.2 | 185 Onions | 10.0 | 78.9 | 1.4.| 0.3| 8.9| 0.5 | 190 Parsnips | 20.0 | 66.4 | 1.3.| 0.4| 10.8| 1.1 | 230 Peas (Pisum sativum), | | | | | | | dried. | -- | 9.5 | 24.6 | 1.0| 62.0| 2.9 | 1565 shelled | -- | 74.6 | 7.0 | 0.5| 16.9| 1.0 | 440 Cowpeas, dried | -- | 13.0 | 21.4.| 1.4| 60.8| 3.4 | 1505 Potatoes | 20.0 | 62.6 | 1.8.| 0.1| 14.7| 0.8 | 295 Vegetables: | | | | | | | Rhubarb | 40.0 | 56.6 | 0.4 | 0.4 | 2.2| 0.4 | 60 Sweet potatoes | 20.0 | 55.2 | 1.4 | 0.6| 21.9| 0.9 | 440 Spinach | -- | 92.3 | 2.1 | 0.3 | 3.2| 2.1 | 95 Squash | 50.0 | 44.2 | 0.7 | 0.2 | 4.5| 0.4 | 100 Tomatoes | -- | 94.3 | 0.9 | 0.4 | 3.9| 0.5 | 100 Turnips | 30.0 | 62.7 | 0.9 | 0.1 | 5.7| 0.6 | 120 Vegetables, canned: | | | | | | | Baked beans | -- | 68.9 | 6.9 | 2.5 | 19.6| 2.1 | 555 Peas (Pisum sativum), | | | | | | green | -- | 85.3 | 3.6 | 0.2 | 9.8| 1.1 | 235 Corn, green | -- | 76.1 | 2.8 | 1.2 | 19.0| 0.9 | 430 Succotash | -- | 75.9 | 3.6 | 1.0 | 18.6| 0.9 | 425 Tomatoes | -- |

94.0 | 1.2 | 0.2 | 4.0| 0.6 | 95 Fruits, berries, etc., | | | | | | | fresh: [E] | | | | | | |
Apples | 25.0 | 63.3 | 0.3 | 0.3 | 10.8| 0.3 | 190 Bananas | 35.0 | 48.9 | 0.8 | 0.4
| 14.3| 0.6 | 260 Grapes | 25.0 | 58.0 | 1.0 | 1.2 | 14.4| 0.4 | 295 Lemons | 30.0 |
62.5 | 0.7 | 0.5 | 5.9| 0.4 | 125 Muskmelons | 50.0 | 44.8 | 0.3 | -- | 4.6| 0.3 | 80
Oranges | 27.0 | 63.4 | 0.6 | 0.1 | 8.5| 0.4 | 150 Pears | 10.0 | 76.0 | 0.5 | 0.4 |
12.7| 0.4 | 230 Persimmons, edible portion | -- | 66.1 | 0.8 | 0.7 | 31.5| 0.9 |
550 Raspberries | -- | 85.8 | 1.0 | -- | 12.6| 0.6 | 220 Strawberries | 5.0 | 85.9 |
0.9 | 0.6 | 7.0| 0.6 | 150 Watermelons | 59.4 | 37.5 | 0.2 | 0.1 | 2.7| 0.1 | 50
Fruits, dried: | | | | | | | Apples | -- | 28.1 | 1.6 | 2.2 | 66.1| 2.0 | 1185 Apricots | -
- | 29.4 | 4.7 | 1.0 | 62.5| 2.4 | 1125 Dates | 10.0 | 13.8 | 1.9 | 2.5 | 70.6| 1.2 |
1275 Fruits, dried: | | | | | | | Rhubarb | 40.0 | 56.6 | 0.4 | 0.4 | 2.2| 0.4 | 60 | | | | |
| | Figs | -- | 18.8 | 4.3 | 0.3 | 74.2| 2.4 | 1280 Raisins | 10.0 | 13.1 | 2.3 | 3.0 |
68.5| 3.1 | 1265 Nuts: | | | | | | | | Almonds | 45.0 | 2.7 | 11.5 | 30.2 | 9.5| 1.1 |
1515 Brazil nuts | 49.6 | 2.6 | 8.6 | 33.7 | 3.5| 2.0 | 1485 Butternuts | 86.4 | 0.6
| 3.8 | 8.3 | 0.5| 0.4 | 385 Chestnuts, fresh | 16.0 | 37.8 | 5.2 | 4.5 | 35.4| 1.1 |
915 Chestnuts, dried | 24.0 | 4.5 | 8.1 | 5.3 | 56.4| 1.7 | 1385 Cocoanuts [F]|
48.8 | 7.2 | 2.9 | 25.9 | 14.3| 0.9 | 1295 Cocoanut, prepared | -- | 3.5 | 6.3 | 57.4
| 31.5| 1.3 | 2865 Filberts | 52.1 | 1.8 | 7.5 | 31.3 | 6.2| 1.1 | 1430 Hickory nuts
| 62.2 | 1.4 | 5.8 | 25.5 | 4.3| 0.8 | 1145 Pecans, polished | 53.2 | 1.4 | 5.2 | 33.3
| 6.2| 0.7 | 1465 Peanuts | 24.5 | 6.9 | 19.5 | 29.1 | 18.5| 1.5 | 1775 Pin (Pinus
edulis) | 40.6 | 2.0 | 8.7 | 36.8 | 10.2| 1.7 | 1730 Walnuts, black | 74.1 | 0.6 |
7.2 | 14.6 | 3.0| 0.5 | 730 Walnuts, English | 58.1 | 1.0 | 6.9 | 26.6 | 6.8| 0.6 |
1250 Miscellaneous: | | | | | | | Chocolate | -- | 5.9 | 12.9 | 48.7 | 30.3| 2.2 | 5625
Cocoa, powdered | -- | 4.6 | 21.6 | 28.9 | 37.7| 7.2 | 2160 Cereal coffee,
infusion | | | | | | | (1 part boiled in | | | | | | | 20 parts water)[G] | -- | 98.2 | 0.2 | -
-          | 1.4| 0.2 | 30

===

============================

[Footnote A: Refuse, oil.] [Footnote B: Refuse, shell.]

[Footnote C: Plain confectionery not containing nuts, fruit, or chocolate.]

[Footnote D: Such vegetables as potatoes, squash, beets, etc., have a certain amount of inedible material, skin, seeds, etc The amount varies with the method of preparing the vegetables, and cannot be accurately estimated The figures given for refuse of vegetables, fruits, etc., are assumed to represent approximately the amount of refuse in these foods as ordinarily prepared.]

[Footnote E: Fruits contain a certain proportion of inedible materials, as skin, seeds, etc., which are properly classed as refuse. In some fruits, as oranges and prunes, the amount rejected in eating is practically the same as refuse. In others, as apples and pears, more or less of the edible material is ordinarily rejected with the skin and seeds and other inedible portions. The edible material which is thus thrown away, and should properly be classed with the waste, is here classed with the refuse. The figures for refuse here given represent, as nearly as can be ascertained, the quantities ordinarily rejected.]

[Footnote F: Milk and shell.]

[Footnote G: The average of five analyses of cereal coffee grain is: Water 6.2, protein 13.3, fat 3.4, carbohydrates 72.6, and ash 4.5 per cent. Only a portion of the nutrients, however, enter into the infusion. The average in the table represents the available nutrients in the beverage. Infusions of genuine coffee and of tea like the above contain practically no nutrients.]

CHAPTER XVII

DIETARY STUDIES

244. Object of Dietary Studies.--The quantity of food which different families purchase varies between wide limits; a portion being lost mechanically in preparation and a still larger and more variable amount in the refuse and non-edible parts. If a record is made of all foods purchased and the waste and non-edible portions are deducted, the nutrients consumed by a family may be calculated by multiplying the weight of each food by the average composition. If such calculations be made, it will be found that in

some families nearly a half pound per day of both protein and fat is consumed by adults, while in other families less than half of this amount is used. The object of dietary studies is to determine the source, cost, composition, and nutritive value of the foods consumed by different families; they also enable comparisons to be made of the amounts of nutrients purchased. Extensive dietary studies have been made by the United States Department of Agriculture, and the results have been published in various bulletins.[76]

245. Wide and Narrow Rations.--When the amount of carbohydrates in a ration is small in comparison with the protein, it is called a narrow ration, while a wide ration is one in which the carbohydrates are much in excess of the protein. When a ration contains 0.40 of a pound of protein, 0.40 of a pound of fat, and 1 pound of carbohydrates, it has a nutritive ratio of 1 to 4.8 and is a narrow ration. To calculate the nutritive ratio, the fat is multiplied by 2-1/4, the product added to the carbohydrates, and this sum divided by the protein. It is not possible to designate accurately the amount of protein and other nutrients that should be in the daily ration of all persons, because the needs of the body vary so with different individuals. Hard and fast rules governing the amounts of nutrients to be consumed cannot as yet be formulated, as our knowledge of the subject is too limited. It is known that both excessive and scant amounts are alike injurious. While the appetite may indicate either hunger or satiety, it alone cannot always be relied upon as a safe guide for determining the amount and kind of food to consume, although the demands of appetite should not be disregarded until it has been demonstrated beyond a doubt that it is not voicing the needs of nature. There has been a tendency which perhaps was a survival of the Puritanical ideas of the early days to stamp as hurtful whatever seemed desirable and pleasant; as examples might be cited the craving for water by fever patients, and for sugar by growing children, which have now been proven to be normal demands of nature.

246. Dietary Standards.--As a result of a large number of dietary studies and digestion experiments, dietary standards have been prepared. Atwater in

this country and Voit in Germany have proposed such standards for men employed at different kinds of labor, as follows:

	Protein lb.	Fat lb.	Carbo-hydrates lb.	Fuel Value Calories	Nutritive Ratio
Man with little physical exercise	0.20	0.20	0.66	2450	5.5
Man with light muscular work	0.22	0.22	0.77	2800	5.7
Man with moderate muscular work	0.28	0.28	0.99	3520	5.8
Man with active muscular work	0.33	0.33	1.10	4060	5.6
Man with hard muscular work	0.39	0.55	1.43	5700	6.9

In the table it will be seen that the quantity of nutrients increases with the labor to be performed. In order to secure the necessary heat and energy, rations for men at heavy labor contain proportionally more fat and carbohydrates than are required for light work. All dietary standards, however, should be regarded as tentative only. Opinions differ greatly on different points; for example, as to the amount of protein a ration should contain. This is a matter that can be determined only from extended investigations under a variety of conditions, and as yet results are too meager to formulate other than tentative standards. Chittenden has found that the body can be sustained on very much less protein than is called for in the standard ration.[77] The amount of protein in the ration should be ample to sustain the body weight and maintain a nitrogen equilibrium; that is, the income and outgo of nitrogen from the body should be practically equal.

(From Office of Experiment Stations Bulletin.)]

"While one freely admits that health and a large measure of muscular strength may be maintained upon a minimum supply of protein, yet I think that a dispassionate survey of mankind will show that races which adopt such a diet are lacking in what, for want of a better word, one can only describe as energy." [28]

On the other hand, excessive and unnecessarily large amounts of protein are sometimes consumed, adding greatly to the cost of the ration and necessitating additional labor on the part of the body for its elimination.

247. Number of Meals per Day.--Some persons advocate two meals per day rather than three, but dietary studies show that the best results are secured when the food is divided among three rather than two meals, and with a two-meal system the tendency is to consume a larger total amount of food than when three meals are eaten. It is not essential that the food be equally divided among the three meals. Any one of them may be lighter or more substantial as the habits and inclinations of the individual dictate. If it is found necessary to reduce the total quantity of food consumed, this may be done by a proportional reduction of each of the meals, or of any one of them instead of decreasing the number of meals per day. The occasional missing of a meal is sometimes beneficial, in cases of digestion disorders, but the ordinary requirements of persons in normal health who have either mental or physical labor to perform are best met when three meals per day are consumed, as this insures an even supply of nutrients. For persons of sedentary habits, the kind and quantity of food at each meal must be regulated largely by the individual from knowledge based on personal experience.

"In the matter of diet every man must, in the last resort, be a law unto himself; but he should draw up his dietetic code intelligently and apply it honestly, giving due heed to the warnings which nature is sure to address to him should he at any time transgress."[28]

If there is trouble in digesting the food, it is well to study the other habits of life along with the food question, for it may be the difficulty arises from some other cause, and would be remedied by more exercise and fresh air, avoiding rush immediately after meals, more thorough mastication, or less worry. It is a serious matter to shut off the supply of food from a person not suffering from some disease and who is working; as well cut off the supply of fuel from a furnace and then expect a full amount of energy and heat. But unlike the furnace, when the human body is deprived of needed nutrients it preys upon itself and uses up its reserve that should be drawn upon only in cases of illness or extreme nervous strain. Some persons live in such a way as to never have any reserve of strength and energy to call upon but use up each day all the body can produce and so become physical bankrupts when they should be in their prime. Food is required for the production of nerve energy as well as physical energy.[78]

248. Mixed Dietary Desirable.--Experiments in the feeding of farm animals show that the best results come from the combination of a number of foods to form a mixed ration, rather than from the use of one food alone,[79] for in this way the work of digestion is more evenly distributed, and a higher degree of efficiency is secured from the foods consumed. The same is true in human feeding; the best results are secured from a mixed diet. Ordinarily, about two fifths of the nutrients of a ration are derived from animal and three fifths from vegetable sources.

249. Animal and Vegetable Foods; Economy of Production.--Animal foods can never compete in cheapness of the nutrients with cereals and vegetables, as it takes six to eight pounds or more of a cereal, together with forage crops, to make a pound of meat. Hence the returns in food value are very much larger from the direct use of the cereals as human food, than from the feeding of cereals to cattle and the use of the meat. As the population of a country increases, and foods necessarily become more expensive, cereals are destined to replace animal foods to a great extent, solely as a matter of economy.

250. Food Habits.--Long-established dietary habits and customs are not easily changed, and when the body becomes accustomed to certain foods, substitution of others, although equally valuable, may fail to give satisfactory results. For example, immigrants from southern Europe demand

foods with which they are familiar, as macaroni, olive oil, and certain kinds of cheese, foods which are generally imported and more expensive than the staples produced in this country,[80] and when they are compelled to live on other foods, even though they have as many nutrients, they complain of being underfed. Previously acquired food habits appear to affect materially the process of digestion and assimilation. Sudden and pronounced change in the feeding of farm animals is attended with unsatisfactory results, and whenever changes are made in the food of either humans or animals they should be gradual rather than radical.

251. Underfed Families.--As the purchasing of food is often done by inexperienced persons, palatability rather than nutritive value is made the basis of choice. Dietary studies show that because of lack of knowledge of the nutritive value of foods, whole families are often underfed. Particularly is this true where the means for purchasing foods are limited. In dietary studies among poor families in New York City,[81] the United States Department of Agriculture notes: "It is quite evident that what is needed among these families more than anything else is instruction in the way to make the little they have go the farthest." Some classes of the rich too are equally liable to be underfed, as they are more prone to food notions and are able to indulge them. Among the children of the rich are found some as poorly nourished as among the poor.

252. Cheap and Expensive Foods.--Among the more expensive items of a ration are meats, butter, and canned fruits. The difference in composition and nutritive value between various cuts of meat is small, being largely physical, and affecting taste and flavor rather than nutritive value. Expensive cuts of meat, high-priced breakfast cereals, tropical fruits and foods which impart special flavors, add little in the way of nutritive value to the ration, but greatly enhance the cost of living. Ordinarily the cheapest foods are corn meal, wheat flour and bread, milk, beans, cheese, sugar, and potatoes.[7] The amount of animal and vegetable foods to combine with these to form a balanced ration may be governed largely by personal preference or cost, as there is little difference in nutritive value. The selection of foods on the basis

of cost and nutritive value is discussed in Chapter XVI.

253. Food Notions.--Many erroneous ideas exist as to the nutritive value of foods, and often wholesome and valuable foods are discriminated against because of prejudice. Skim milk is usually regarded as containing little if any nourishing material, when in reality it has a high protein content, and can be added to other foods to increase their nutritive value. The less expensive cuts of meat contain more total nutrients than many of the more expensive ones. Beef extracts have been erroneously said to contain more nutrients than beef,[51] and mushrooms to be equal in value of beefsteak; chemical analyses fail to confirm either statement. The banana also has been overestimated as to food value, and while it contains more nutrients than many fruits, it is not the equal of cereals, as has been claimed.[82] Cocoa, although a valuable beverage, adds but little in the way of nutrients to a ration unless it is made with milk. The value of a food should be based upon its composition as determined by chemical analysis, its digestibility as founded upon digestion experiments, and its palatability and mechanical structure. Food notions have, in many instances, been the cause of banishing from the dietary wholesome and nutritious foods, of greatly increasing the cost of living, as well as of promulgating incorrect ideas in regard to foods, so that individuals and in some cases entire families have suffered from improper or insufficient food.

254. Dietary of Two Families Compared.--A dietary study often reveals ways in which it is possible to improve the ration in kinds and amounts of food, and sometimes at less expense. The following dietaries of two families for the same period show that one family expends over twice as much in the purchase of foods as the other family, and yet the one whose food costs the less actually secures the larger amount of nutritive material and is better fed than the family where more money is expended for food.[13]

FOOD CONSUMED, ONE WEEK

FAMILY No. 1

20 loaves of bread $1.00 10 to 12 lb. loin steak, or meat of similar cost 2.00 20 to 25 lb. rib roast, or similar meat 4.40 4 lb. high-priced cereal breakfast food, 20 ct. 0.80 Cake and pastry purchased 3.00 8 lb. butter, 30 ct. 2.40 Tea, coffee, spices, etc 0.75 Mushrooms 0.75 Celery 1.00 Oranges 2.00 Potatoes 0.25 Miscellaneous canned goods 2.00 Milk 0.50 Miscellaneous foods 2.00 3 doz. eggs 0.60 ------ $23.45

FAMILY No. 2

15 lb. flour, bread home-made (skim milk used) $0.45 Yeast, shortening and skim milk 0.10 10 lb. steak (round. Hamburger and some loin) 1.50 10 lb. other meats, boiling pieces, rump roast, etc. 1.00 5 lb. cheese, 16 cents 0.80 5 lb. oatmeal (bulk) 0.15 5 lb. beans 0.25 Home-made cake and pastry 1.00 6 lb. butter, 30 ct. 1.80 3 lb. home-made shortening 0.25 Tea, coffee, and spices 0.40 Apples 0.50 Prunes 0.25 Potatoes 0.25 Milk 1.00 Miscellaneous foods 1.00 3 doz. eggs 0.60 ------ $11.30

In comparing the foods used by the two families, it will be observed that family No. 1 purchased their bread at the bakery at a cost of $ 1.00, while the bread of family No. 2 was home-made, skim milk being used in its preparation, the flour, milk, yeast, and shortening costing about 55 cents. Family No. 1 consumed 10 pounds of expensive steaks, family No. 2 consumed the same number of pounds, a portion being cheaper cuts. Instead of the 20 pounds of roast or similar beef used by family No. 1, only one half as much and cheaper cuts as boiling pieces, stew, rump roast, etc., were used by family No. 2; 5 pounds of beans and 5 pounds of cheese taking the place of some of the meat. Family No. 1 consumed 4 pounds of high-priced cereal breakfast foods, supposing they contained a larger amount of nutrients than were actually present. In place of the 4 pounds of high-priced cereal breakfast foods of family No. 1, family No. 2 used 5 pounds of oatmeal purchased in bulk. Family No. 1 bought their cake and pastry for $3.00, while those of family No. 2 were home made and cost $1.00. Family No. 2 used 2 pounds less butter per week because of the preparation and use of home-made shortening from beef suet and milk. They also purchased a smaller amount of tea, coffee, and spices than family No. 1. Family No. 2 consumed a larger quantity of less expensive fruits and vegetables than family No. 1, who ate 75 cents' worth of mushrooms with the idea that they contained as much protein as meat, but analyses show that mushrooms contain no more nutrients than potatoes and similar vegetables. In place of the celery and oranges, apples and prunes were used by family No. 2. The same amount of potatoes was used by each. Fifty cents was spent for milk by family No. 1 and $1.00 by family No. 2. The total amount expended for food by family No. 1 was $23.45, while family No. 2 purchased a greater variety of foods for $11.30, as well as foods containing more nutrients. The approximate amounts of nutrients in the foods purchased by the two families are given in the following table, from which it will be observed that family No. 2 obtained a much larger amount of total nutrients and was better fed at considerably less expense than family No. 1.

NUTRIENTS IN FOODS CONSUMED.--FAMILY NO. 1

	PROTEIN LB.	FAT LB.	CARBOHYDRATES LB.
20 lb. bread	1.98	0.28	11.42
10 lb. loin steak	1.59	1.76	--
20 lb. rib roast	2.68	4.26	--
4 lb. cereals	0.42	0.06	2.75
8 lb. butter	0.04	6.80	--
25 lb. potatoes	0.45	0.03	3.83
20 lb. milk	0.70	0.80	1.00
	7.86	13.99	19.00

FAMILY NO. 2

	PROTEIN LB.	FAT LB.	CARBOHYDRATES LB.
15 lb. flour	1.89	0.12	11.15
5 lb. skim milk	0.16	0.01	0.26
10 lb. round steak	1.81	1.26	--
10 lb. beef	1.32	2.02	--
5 lb. cheese	1.40	1.75	--
5 lb. oatmeal	0.78	0.36	3.40
6 lb. butter	0.03	5.10	--
3 lb. shortening	--	2.55	--
3 lb. prunes	0.03	--	0.60
25 lb. apples	0.12	--	2.50
25 lb. potatoes	0.45	0.03	3.83
40 lb. milk	1.44	1.60	

```
1.90 5 lb. beans | 1.12 | -- | 3.00 ------------------------|-------|-----|---------------
--- | 10.55 |14.80| 26.64  ------------------------|-------|-----|-----------------
Difference in nutrients | in favor of family No. 2,| consuming the cheaper
|2.69      0.81      7.64         combination      of       foods       |
================================================================
```

255. Food in its Relation to Mental and Physical Vigor.--When the body is not properly supplied with food, the best results in the form of productive work cannot be secured. There is a close relationship between the nature of the food consumed and mental activity, also ability to satisfactorily perform physical labor. "The productive power of the individual as well as of the nation depends doubtless upon many factors other than food, such as race, climate, habit, etc., but there is no gainsaying the fact that diet has also a profound and direct influence upon it."[83]

If the body is diseased, it cannot make the right uses of the food, and often the food is blamed when the trouble is due primarily to other causes. The fact that a diseased digestive tract is unable to utilize some foods is no valid reason why these foods should be discarded in the dietary of persons in normal health, particularly when the food is in no way responsible for the disease.

Some diseases are most prevalent in the case of a restricted diet. A change in the dietary of the Japanese navy greatly improved the health of the sailors.

"The prevalence of kakke or beriberi in the navy turned the attention of many medical specialists toward the problem of nutrition.... It was generally believed that there was some very close connection between the disease and the rice diet.... One outcome of these investigations was the passage of the food supply act of the navy in 1884. The ration provided in accordance with this act was sufficient to furnish an abundance of protein and energy.... Following the change of ration in 1884, the prevalence of the disease was very materially diminished, and at the end of three years cases of kakke were practically unknown among the marines."[83]

256. Dietary Studies in Public Institutions.--Dietary studies in public institutions, as prisons, and asylums for the insane, show that it is possible to secure greater variety of food containing a larger amount of nutrients, and even at a reduction in cost.[84] In such institutions it is important that the food should be not only ample in amount, but wholesome and nutritious, as many of the inmates respond both physically and mentally to an improved diet. For humanitarian as well as economic reasons institutional dietetics should more generally be placed under the supervision of skilled dietists.

CHAPTER XVIII

RATIONAL FEEDING OF MAN

257. Object.--Rational feeding of man has for its object the regulation of the food supply in accord with the demands of the body. It is based upon the same principles as the rational feeding of animals; in each, the best results in the way of health, amount of labor performed, and economy are secured when the body receives nutrients sufficient for the production of heat and energy and for the repair of worn-out tissues. Rational feeding is simply regulation of the food, both as to kind and amount, to meet the needs of the body.[72]

258. Standard Rations.--In human feeding, as in animal feeding, it is not possible to lay down hard and fast rules as to the quantity of nutrients required for a standard ration.[85] As stated in the chapter on Dietary Studies, such standards have been proposed, but they are to be considered as tentative rather than absolute, for the amount of food required by different persons must necessarily vary with the individuality. While it is impossible to establish absolute standards, any large variation from the provisional standards usually results in lessened ability to accomplish work, ill health, or increased expense.

259. Amounts of Food Consumed.--The approximate amounts of some

food articles consumed per day are as follows:

```
============================================   |     RANGE     |
APPROXIMATE | |AMOUNT IN LBS. --------|------------------------- Bread
|6 to 14 oz.| 0.50 Butter |2 to 5 oz.| 0.12 Potatoes|8 to 16 oz.| 0.75 Cheese |1
to 4 oz.| 0.12 Beans |1 to 4 oz.| 0.12 Milk |8 to 32 oz.| -- Sugar |2 to 5 oz.|
0.20  Meats  |4  to  12  oz.|  0.25  Oatmeal  |1  to  4  oz.|  0.12
=====================================
```

In the calculation of rations it is desirable that the amount of any food article should not exceed that designated, unless for some special reason it has been found the food can consistently be increased. The amount of nutrients given in dietary standards is for one day, and the nutrients may be divided among the three meals as desired. It is to be noted that, ordinarily, the foods which supply carbohydrates are flour, corn meal, cereal products, potatoes, beans, sugar, and milk; those which supply fat are milk, butter, lard, and meats; and those which supply protein in liberal amounts are beans, cheese, meats, oatmeal, cereals, bread, and milk.

260. Average Composition of Foods.--The amounts of nutrients in foods are determined from the average composition of the foods. These figures for average composition are based upon analyses of a large number of samples of food materials.[7] In individual cases it will be found that foods may vary from the standards given; as for example, milk may contain from 2.5 to 5 per cent of fat, while the protein and fat of meats vary appreciably from the figures given for average composition. With the cereals and vegetable foods, variations from the standards are small. In the table, the composition of the food as purchased represents all of the nutrients in the food, including those in the refuse, trimmings, or waste, while the figures for the edible portion represent the nutrients in the food after deducting what is lost as refuse. In making calculations, the student should use the figures given for the foods as purchased, unless the weights are of the edible portion only. The figures in the table are on the basis of percentage amounts, or nutrients in 100 pounds of food. By moving the decimal point two places to the left, the figures will

represent the nutrients in one pound, and if this is multiplied by the number of pounds or fraction of a pound used, the quantity of nutrients is secured. For example, suppose bread contains 9.5 per cent of protein and 56 per cent of carbohydrates, 1 pound would contain 0.095 pound of protein, 0.56 pound of carbohydrates; and 0.5 of a pound would contain approximately 0.05 pound of protein and 0.28 pound of carbohydrates. In calculating rations, it is not necessary to carry the figures to the third decimal place.

261. Example of a Ration.--Suppose it is desired to calculate a ration for a man at light muscular work. First, note the requirements in the way of nutrients in the table "Dietary Standards," Section 246. Such a ration should supply approximately 0.22 pound each of protein and fat, and 0.77 pound of carbohydrates, and should yield 2800 calories. A trial ration is made by combining the following:

```
========================================================================
===== | Pound Bread | 0.50 Butter | 0.12 Potatoes | 0.75 Milk | 1.00 Sugar |
0.12  Beef  |  0.25  Ham  |  0.20  Oatmeal  |  0.12  Eggs  |  0.25
========================================================================
=====
```

The quantities of nutrients in these food materials are approximately as follows:

RATION FOR MAN AT MODERATE WORK

```
========================================================================
============== | | PROTEIN | FAT | C.H. | | LB. | LB. | LB. | LB. |
CALORIES      -------------------------+------+---------+------+------+----------
Bread | 0.50 | 0.05 | 0.01 | 0.29 | 653 Butter | 0.12 | -- | 0.10 | -- | 432 Potato |
0.75 | 0.01 | -- | 0.12 | 244 Milk | 1.00 | 0.04 | 0.04 | 0.05 | 323 Sugar | 0.12 | --
| -- | 0.12 | 192 Beef (round) | 0.25 | 0.05 | 0.03 | -- | 218 Ham | 0.20 | 0.03 |
```

```
0.07 | -- | 331 Oatmeal | 0.12 | 0.02 | 0.01 | 0.08 | 223 Eggs | 0.25 | 0.03 | 0.03
| -- | 164 Squash | 0.20 | -- | -- | 0.01 | 25 |------+---------+------+------+----------
|      |      0.23      |      0.29      |      0.67      |      2805
============================================================================
===============
```

It is to be noted that this ration contains approximately the amount of protein called for in the standard ration, while the fat is slightly more and the carbohydrates are less. The food value of the ration is practically that called for in the standard. This ration is sufficiently near the standard to supply the nutrient requirements of a man at light muscular work. To supply palatability, some fruit and vegetables should be added to the ration. These will contribute but little to the nutrient content, but are necessary in order to secure health and the best returns from the other foods, and as previously stated, they are not to be estimated entirely upon the basis of nutrient content. A number of food articles could be substituted in this ration, if desired, either in the interests of economy, palatability, or personal preference.

262. Requisites of a Balanced Ration.--Reasonable combinations of foods should be made to form balanced rations.[2] A number of foods slow of digestion, or which require a large amount of intestinal work, should not be combined; neither should foods which are easily digested and which leave but little indigestible residue. After a ration has been calculated and found to contain the requisite amount of nutrients, it should be critically examined to see whether or not it fulfills the following requirements:

1. Economy and adaptability to the work required.

2. Necessary bulk or volume.

3. Desired physiological influence of the foods upon the digestive tract, whether constipating or laxative in character.

4. Ease of digestion.

5. Effect upon health. It is recognized that there are foods wholesome and nutritious, that cannot be used by some persons, while with others the same foods can be consumed with impunity.

As explained in the chapter on Dietary Studies, the nutrients should be supplied from a number of foods rather than from a few, because it is believed the various nutrients, particularly the proteins, are not absolutely identical from all sources, or equal in nutritive value.

EXAMPLES

1. Calculate a ration for a man with little physical exercise.

2. Calculate a ration for a man at hard muscular labor, and give the approximate cost of the ration.

3. Calculate the amounts of food and the nutrient requirements for a family of seven for 10 days; five of the family to consume 0.8 as much as an adult. Calculate the cost of the food; then calculate on the same basis the probable cost of food for one year, adding 20 per cent for fluctuation in market price and additional foods not included in the list.

4. Weigh out the food articles used in problem No. 2, and apportion them among three meals.

CHAPTER XIX

WATER

263. Importance.--Water is one of the most essential food materials. It enters into the composition of the body, and without it the nutrients of foods would be unavailable, and life could not be sustained. Water unites chemically with various elements to form plant tissue and supplies hydrogen

and oxygen for the production of organic compounds within the leaves of plants. In the animal economy it is not definitely known whether or not water furnishes any of the elements of which the tissues are composed, as the food contains liberal amounts of hydrogen and oxygen; it is necessary mainly as the vehicle for distributing nutrients in suspension and solution, and as a medium in which chemical, physical, and physiological changes essential to life processes take place. From a sanitary point of view, the condition of the water supply is of great importance, as impure water seriously affects the health of the consumer.[87]

264. Impurities in Water.--Waters are impure because of: (1) excessive amounts of alkaline salts and other mineral compounds; (2) decaying animal and vegetable matters which act chemically as poisons and irritants, and which may serve as food for the development of objectionable bacterial bodies; and (3) injurious bacteria. The most common forms of impurities are excess of organic matter and bacterial contamination. The sanitary condition of water is greatly influenced by the character of the soil through which it flows and the extent to which it has been polluted by surface drainage.[88]

265. Mineral Impurities.--- The mineral impurities of water are mainly soluble alkaline and similar compounds dissolved by the water in passing through various layers of soil and rock. When water contains a large amount of sodium chloride, sodium sulphate or carbonate, or other alkaline salts, it is termed an "alkali water." Where water passes through soil that has been largely formed from the decay of rocks containing alkaline minerals, the water dissolves some of these minerals and becomes alkaline. The kind of alkali determines the character of the water; in some cases it is sodium carbonate, which is particularly objectionable. The continued use of strong alkali water causes digestion disorders, because of the irritating action upon the digestive tract. Hard waters are due to the presence of lime compounds. In regions where limestone predominates, the carbon dioxid in water acts as a solvent, producing hard waters. Waters that are hard on account of the presence of calcium carbonate give a deposit when boiled, due to liberation of the carbon dioxid which is the material that renders the lime soluble.

Calcium sulphate, or gypsum, on the other hand, imparts permanent hardness. There is no deposit when such waters are boiled. A large number of minerals are found in various waters, often sufficient in amount to impart physiological properties. Water that is highly charged with mineral matter is difficult to improve sufficiently for household purposes. About the only way is by distillation.[89]

266. Organic Impurities.--Water that flows over the surface of the ground comes in contact with animal and vegetable material in various stages of decay, and as a result some is dissolved and some is mechanically carried along by the water. After becoming soluble, the organic matter undergoes further chemical changes, as oxidation and nitrification caused by bacteria. If the organic matter contain a large amount of nitrogenous material, particularly of proteid origin, a series of chemical changes induced by bacterial action takes place, resulting in the production of nitrites. The nitrifying organisms first produce nitrous acid products (nitrites), and in the further development of the nitrifying process these are changed to nitrates. The ammonia formed as the result of the decomposition of nitrogenous organic matter readily undergoes nitrification changes. Nitrates and nitrites alone are not injurious in water, but they are usually associated with objectionable bacteria and generally indicate previous contamination.[90]

267. Interpretation of a Water Analysis.--"Total solid matter" represents all the mineral, vegetable, and animal matter which a water contains. It is the residue obtained by evaporating the water to dryness at a temperature of 212?F. Average drinking water contains from 20 to 90 grains per gallon of solid matter. "Free ammonia" is that formed as a result of the decomposition of animal or vegetable matter containing nitrogen. Water of high purity usually contains less than 0.07 parts per million of free ammonia. "Albuminoid ammonia" is derived from the partially decomposed animal or vegetable material in water. The greater the amount of nitrogenous organic impurities, the higher the albuminoid ammonia. A good drinking water ought not to contain more than 0.10 part per million of albuminoid ammonia. An abnormal quantity of chlorine indicates surface drainage or sewage

contamination, or an excess of alkaline matter, as common salt. Nitrites should not be present, as they are generally associated with matter not completely oxidized. Nitrites are usually considered more objectionable than nitrates; both are innocuous unless associated with disease-producing nitroorganisms.

268. Natural Purification of Water.--River waters are sometimes dark colored because of large amounts of dissolved organic matter, but in contact with the sun and air they gradually undergo natural purification and the organic matter is oxidized. However, absolute reliance cannot be placed upon natural purification of a bad water, as the objectionable organisms often have great resistive power. There is no perfectly pure water except that prepared in the chemical laboratory by distillation. All natural waters come in contact with the soil and air, and necessarily contain impurities proportional to the extent of their contamination.

269. Water in Relation to Health.--There are many diseases, of which typhoid fever is a type, that are distinctly water-born. The typhoid bacilli, present in countless numbers in the feces of persons suffering or convalescent from typhoid fever, find their way into streams, lakes, and wells.[91] They retain their vitality, and when they enter the digestive tract of an individual, rapidly increase in numbers. Numerous disastrous outbreaks of typhoid fever have been traced to contamination of water. Coupled with the sanitary improvement of a city's water supply, there is diminution of typhoid fever cases, and a noticeable lowering of the death rate. Many cities and villages are dependent for their water upon rivers and lakes into which surface drainage finds its way, with all contaminating substances. Mechanical sedimentation and filtration greatly improve waters of this class, but do not necessarily render them entirely pure. Compounds of iron and aluminium are sometimes added in small amounts, under chemical supervision, to such waters to precipitate the organic impurities. Spring waters are not entirely above suspicion, as oftentimes the soil through which they flow is highly polluted. All water of doubtful purity should be boiled, and there are but few natural waters of undoubted purity. There is no such

thing as absolutely pure water in a state of nature. The mountain streams perhaps approach nearest to it where there are no humans to pollute the banks; but then there are always the beasts and birds, and they, too, are subject to disease. There are very few waters that at some time of the year and under some conditions are not contaminated with disease-producing organisms. No matter how carefully guarded are the banks of lakes furnishing the water supply of cities, more or less objectionable matter will get in. In seasons of heavy rains, large amounts of surface water enter the lakes, carrying along the filth gathered from many acres of land drained by the streams entering the lakes. Some of the most serious outbreaks of typhoid fever have come from temporary contamination of ordinarily fairly good drinking water. In general, too little attention is given to the purity of drinking water. It is just as important that water should be boiled as that food should be cooked. One of the objects of cooking is to destroy the injurious bacteria, and they are frequently more numerous in the drinking water than in the food.

The argument is sometimes advanced that the mineral matter present in water is needed for the construction of the bone and other tissues of the body, and that distilled water fails to supply the necessary mineral matter. This is an erroneous assumption, as the mineral matter in the food is more than sufficient for this purpose. When water is highly charged with mineral salts, additional work for their elimination is called for on the part of the organs of excretion, particularly the kidneys; and furthermore, water nearly saturated with minerals cannot exert its full solvent action.

In discussing the immediate benefits resulting from improvement of water, Fuertes says:[92]

"Immediately after the change to the 'four mile intake' at Chicago in 1893, there was a great reduction in typhoid. Lawrence, Mass., showed a great improvement with the setting of the filters in operation in September, 1893; fully half of the deaths in 1894 were among persons known to have used the unfiltered canal water. The conclusion is warranted that for the efficient control of the death rate from typhoid fever it is necessary to have efficient sewerage and drainage, proper methods of living, and pure water. The reason why our large cities, which are all provided with sewerage, have such high death rates is therefore without doubt their continuance of the filthy practice of supplying drinking water which carries in solution and suspension the washings from farms, from the streets, from privies, from pigpens, and the sewage of cities.... And also we should recognize the importance of flies and other winged insects and birds which feed on offal as carriers of bacteria of specific diseases from points of infection to the watersheds, and the consequent washing of newly infected matter into our drinking water by rains."

There is a very close relationship between the surface water and that of shallow wells. A shallow well is simply a reservoir for surface water accumulations. It is stated that, when an improved system of drainage was introduced into a part of London, many of the shallow wells became dry, indicating the source from which they received their supply. Direct subterranean connection between cesspools and wells is often traced in the following way: A small amount of lithium, which gives a distinct flame reaction, and a minute trace of which can be detected with the spectroscope, is placed in the cesspool, and after a short time a lithium reaction is secured from the well water.

Rain water is relied upon in some localities for drinking purposes. That collected in cities and in the vicinity of barns and dwellings contains appreciable amounts of organic impurities. The brown color is due to the impurities, ammonium carbonate being one of these. There are also traces of nitrates and nitrites obtained from the air. When used for drinking, rain water should be boiled.

270. Improvement of Waters.--Waters are improved by: (1) boiling, which destroys the disease-producing organisms; (2) filtration, which removes the materials mechanically suspended in the water; and (3) distillation, which eliminates the impurities in suspension and solution, as well as destroys all

germ life.

271. Boiling Water.--In order to destroy the bacteria that may be in drinking water, it is not sufficient to heat the water or merely let it come to a boil. It has been found that if water is only partially sterilized and then cooled in the open air, the bacteria develop more rapidly than if the water had not been heated at all. It should boil vigorously five to ten minutes; cholera and typhoid bacteria succumb in five minutes or less. Care should be taken in cooling that the water is not exposed to dust particles from the air nor placed in open vessels in a dirty refrigerator. It should be kept in perfectly clean, tight-stoppered bottles. These bottles should be frequently scalded. Great reliance may be placed upon this method of water purification when properly carried out.

272. Filtration.--Among the most efficient forms of water filters are the Berkefeld and Pasteur. The Pasteur filter is made of unglazed porcelain, and the Berkefeld of fine infusorial earth (finely divided $SiO\{2\}$). Both are porous and allow a moderately rapid flow of water. The flow from the Berkefeld filter is more rapid than from the Pasteur. The mechanical impurities of the water are deposited upon the filtering surface, due to the attraction which the material has for particles in suspension. These particles usually are the sources of contamination and carry bacteria. When first used, filters are satisfactory, but unless carefully looked after they soon lose their ability to remove germs from the water and may increase the impurity by accumulation. Small faucet filters are made of porous stone, asbestos, charcoal, etc. Many of them are of no value whatever or are even worse than valueless. Filters should be frequently cleansed in boiling water or in steam under pressure. Unless this is done, the filters may become incubators for bacteria.

273. Distillation.--When an unquestionably pure water supply is desired, distillation should be resorted to. There are many forms of stills for domestic use which are easily manipulated and produce distilled water economically.[93] The mineral matter of water is in no way essential for any

functional purpose, and hence its removal through distillation is not detrimental.

274. Chemical Purification.--Purification of water by the use of chemicals should not be attempted in the household or by inexperienced persons. When done under supervision of a chemist or bacteriologist, it may be of great value to a community. Turneaure and Russell,[94] in discussing the purification of water by addition of chemicals, state:

"There are a considerable number of chemical substances that may be added to water in order to purify it by carrying down the suspended matter as well as bacteria, by sedimentation. Such a process of purification is to be seen in the addition of alum, sulphate of iron, and calcium hydrate to water. Methods of this character are directly dependent upon the flocculating action of the chemical added, and the removal of the bacteria is accomplished by subsidence."

275. Ice.--The purity of the ice supply is also of much importance. While freezing reduces the number of organisms and lessens their vitality, it does not make an impure water absolutely wholesome. The way, too, in which ice is often handled and stored subjects it to contamination, and foods which are placed in direct contact with it mechanically absorb the impurities which it contains. For cooling water, ice should be placed around rather than in it. Diseases have frequently been traced to impure ice. The only absolutely pure ice is that made from distilled water.

276. Mineral Waters.--When water is charged with carbonic acid gas under pressure, carbonated water results, and when minerals, as salts of sodium, potassium, or lithium, are added, artificial mineral waters are produced. Natural mineral waters are placed on the market to some extent, but most mineral waters are artificial products and they are sometimes prepared from water of low sanitary character. Mineral waters should not be used extensively except under medical direction, as many have pronounced medicinal properties. Some of the constituents are bicarbonates of sodium,

potassium, and lithium; sulphates of magnesium (Epsom salts) and calcium; and chloride of sodium. The sweetened mineral waters, as lemonade, orangeade, ginger ale, and beer, contain sugar and organic acids, as citric and tartaric, and are flavored with natural or artificial products. Most of them are prepared without either fruit or ginger. Natural mineral waters used under the direction of a physician are often beneficial in cases of chronic digestion disorders or other diseases.

277. Materials for Softening Water.--The materials most commonly used for softening water are sodium carbonate (washing soda), borax, ammonia, ammonium carbonate, potash, and soda lye. Waters that are very hard with limestone should have a small amount of washing soda added to them. Two ounces for a large tub of water is the most that should be used, and it should first be dissolved in a little water. If too much soda is used, it is injurious, as only a certain amount can be utilized for softening the water, and the excess simply injures the hands and fabric. When hard limewater is boiled and a very little soda lye added, a precipitate of carbonate of lime is formed, and then if the water is strained, it is greatly improved for washing purposes. Borax is valuable for making some hard waters soft. It is not as strong in its action as is sodium carbonate. For the hardest water 1/4 pound of borax to a large tubful may be used; most waters, however, do not need so much. Ammonia is one of the most useful reagents for softening water. It is better than washing soda and borax, because the ammonia is volatile and does not leave any residue to act on the clothes, thus causing injury. For bathing purposes, the water should be softened with ammonia, in preference to any other material. Ammonia should not be poured directly into hot water; it should be added to the water while cold, or to a small quantity of cold water, and then to the warm water, as this prevents the ammonia from vaporizing too readily. Ammonia produces the same effect as potash or soda lye, without leaving a residue in the garments washed. It is especially valuable in washing woolen goods or materials liable to shrink. Waters which are hard with alum salts are greatly benefited by the addition of ammonia. A little in such a water will cause a precipitate to form, and when the water is strained it is in good condition for cleaning purposes. Ammonium carbonate is used

to some extent as a softening and cleaning agent, and is valuable, as there is no injurious effect upon clothing, because it readily volatilizes. Caustic potash and caustic soda are sometimes employed for softening water, but they are very active and are not adapted to washing colored or delicate fabrics. They may be used for very heavy and coarse articles that are greasy,--not more than a gram in a gallon of water. Bleaching powder is not generally a safe material for cleansing purposes, as it weakens the texture of clothing. After a contagious disease, articles may be soaked in water containing a little bleaching powder and a few drops of carbolic acid, followed by thorough rinsing and bleaching in the sun. But as a rule formaline is preferable for disinfecting clothing. It can be used at the rate of about one pound to 100 gallons of water. Bleaching powder, caustic potash or soda, and strong soap are not suitable for cleaning woodwork, because of the action of the alkali on paint and wood; they roughen the surface and discolor the paint. Waters vary so in composition, that a material suitable for softening one may not prove to be the best for softening another. The special kind must be determined largely by trial, and it should be the aim to use as little as possible. When carbolic acid, formaline, bleaching powder, and caustic soda are used, the hands should be protected and the clothes should be well rinsed.

278. Economic Value of a Pure Water Supply.--From a financial point of view, the money spent in securing pure water is one of the best investments a community can make. Statisticians estimate the death of an adult results in a loss to the state of from $1000 to $5000; and to the losses sustained by death must be added those incurred by sickness and by lessened quality and quantity of work through impaired vitality,--all caused by using poor drinking water. Wherever plants have been installed for improving the sanitary condition of the water supply, the death rate has been lowered and the returns to the community have been far greater than the cost of the plant. Impure water is the most expensive food that can be consumed.

CHAPTER XX

FOOD AS AFFECTED BY HOUSEHOLD SANITATION AND STORAGE

279. Injurious Compounds in Foods.--An ordinary chemical analysis of a food determines only the nutrients, as protein, carbohydrates, and fats; and unless there is reason to believe the food contains injurious substances no special tests for these are made. There are a number of poisonous compounds that foods may contain, and many of them can but imperfectly be determined by chemical analysis. Numerous organic compounds are produced in foods as the result of the workings of microoganisms; some of these are poisonous, while others impart only special characteristics, as taste and odor. The poisonous bacteria finding their way into food produce organic compounds of a toxic character; and hence it is that the sanitary condition of a food, as influenced by preparation and storage, is often of more vital importance than the nutrient content.[95]

280. Sources of Contamination of Food.--As a rule, too little attention is given to the sanitary handling and preparation of foods. They are often exposed to impure air and to the dust and filth from unclean streets and surroundings, and as a result they become inoculated with bacteria, which are often the disease-producing kind. Gelatine plates exposed by bacteriologists under the same conditions as foods develop large numbers of injurious microoganisms. In order to avoid contamination in the handling of food, there must be: (1) protection from impure air and dust; (2) storage in clean, sanitary, and ventilated storerooms and warehouses; (3) storage of perishable foods at a low temperature so as to retard fermentation changes; and (4) workmen free from contagious diseases in all occupations pertaining to the preparation of foods. Ordinarily, foods should not be stored in the paper wrappers in which they are purchased, as unclean paper is often a source of contamination.

281. Sanitary Inspection of Food.--During recent years some state and city boards of health have introduced sanitary inspection of foods, with a view of preventing contamination during manufacture and transportation, and this

has done much to improve the quality and wholesomeness. Putrid meats, fish, and vegetables are not allowed to be sold, and foods are required to be handled and stored in a sanitary way. Next to a pure water supply, there is no factor that so greatly influences for good the health of a community as the sanitary condition of the food. While the cooking of foods destroys many organisms, it often fails to render innocuous the poisons which they produce, and furthermore the unsound foods when cooked are not entirely wholesome, and they have poor keeping qualities.

Often meats, vegetables, and other foods eaten uncooked, as well as the numerous cooked foods, are exposed in dirty market places, and accumulate large amounts of filth, and are inoculated with disease germs by flies. Protection of food from flies is a matter of vital importance, as they are carriers of many diseases. In the case of typhoid fever, next to impure drinking water flies are credited with being the greatest distributors of the disease germs.[96]

282. Infection from Impure Air.--The dust particles of the air contain decayed animal and vegetable matter in which bacteria are present; these find their way into the food when it is not carefully protected, into the water supply, and also into the lungs and other organs of the body. When foods are protected from the mechanical impurities which gain access through the air, and fermentation is delayed by storage at a low temperature, digestion disorders are greatly lessened. From a sanitary point of view, the air of food storerooms and of living rooms should be of equally high purity. When foods are kept in unventilated living rooms, they become contaminated with the impurities thrown off from the lungs in respiration, which include not only carbon dioxid, but the more objectionable toxic organic materials.

Vegetable foods need to be stored in well-ventilated places, as the plant cells are still alive and carrying on life functions, as the giving off of carbon dioxid, which is akin to animal respiration; in fact, it is plant-cell respiration. Provision should be made for the removal of the carbon dioxid and other products, as they contaminate the air. When vegetable tissue ceases to produce carbon dioxid, death and decay set in, accompanied by fermentation changes.

283. Storage of Food in Cellars.--Cellars are often in a very unsanitary condition, damp, poorly lighted, unventilated, and the air filled with floating particles from decaying vegetables. The walls and shelves absorb the dust and germs from the foul air and are bacterially contaminated, and whenever a sound food is stored in such a cellar, it readily becomes inoculated with bacteria. There is a much closer relationship existing between the atmosphere of the cellar and that of the house than is generally realized. An unclean cellar means contaminated air throughout the house. When careful attention is given to the sanitary condition of the cellar, many of the more common diseases are greatly reduced. Cases of rheumatism have often been traced to a damp cellar. In some localities where the cellars are unusually unsanitary, there is in the season of spring rains, when they are especially damp and contain the maximum of decayed vegetation, a prevalence of what might be called "cellaritis." The symptoms differ and the trouble is variously attributed, but the real cause is the same, although overlooked, for, unfortunately, doctors do not visit the cellar.

Cellars should be frequently cleaned and disinfected, using for the purpose some of the well-known disinfectants, as formaline, bleaching powder, or a dilute solution of carbolic acid. It has been found in large cities, when the spread of such diseases as yellow fever was imminent, that a general and thorough cleaning up of streets and cellars with the improved sanitary conditions resulting greatly lowered the usual death rate.

284. Sunlight, Pure Water, and Pure Air as Disinfectants.--The most effectual and valuable disinfectants are sunlight, pure water, and pure air. Many kinds of microoganisms, particularly those that are disease-producing, are destroyed when exposed for a time to sunlight. The chemical action of the sun's rays is destructive to the organic material which makes up the composition of many of these organisms, while higher forms of organic life are stirred into activity by it. The disinfecting power of sunlight should be

made use of to the fullest extent, not only in the house, but plenty of sunlight should also be planned for in constructing barns and other buildings where milk-and meat-producing animals are kept. Pure water is also a disinfectant, but when water becomes polluted it loses this power. Many disease-producing organisms are rendered inactive when placed in pure water. Water contains more dissolved oxygen than air, and apparently a portion of the oxygen in water is in a more active condition than that in air. Pure air, too, is a disinfectant; the ozone and hydrogen peroxide and oxides of nitrogen, which are present in traces, exert a beneficial influence in oxidizing organic matter. Fresh air and sunlight, acting jointly, are nature's most effectual disinfectants. Sunshine, fresh air, and pure water are a health-producing trinity. In discussing the importance of pure air, water, and sunlight, Ellen H. Richards[97] says:

"The country dweller surrounds his house with evergreens or shade trees, the city dweller is surrounded with high brick walls. Blinds, shades, or thick draperies shut out still more, and prevent the beneficial sunlight from acting its role of germ prevention and germ destruction. Bright-colored carpets and pale-faced children are the opposite results which follow. Sunlight, pure air, and pure water are our common birthright which we often bargain away for so-called comforts."

And Dr. Woods Hutchinson says of sunlight:

"It is a splendid and matchless servant in the promoting of healthfulness of the house, for which no substitute has yet been discovered. It is the foe alike of bacilli and the blues; the best tonic ever yet invented for the liver and for the scalp, and for everything between, the only real complexion restorer, and the deadliest foe of dirt and disease."

285. Utensils for Storage of Food.--In order that dishes and household utensils may be kept in the best sanitary condition, they should be free from seams, cracks, and crevices where dust and dirt particles can find lodgment. From the seams of a milk pail that has not been well washed, decaying milk

solids can be removed with the aid of a pin or a toothpick. This material acts as a "starter" or culture when pure, fresh milk is placed in the pail, contaminating it and causing it to become sour. Not only is this true of milk, but also of other foods. Wooden utensils are not satisfactory for the handling, storage, or preparation of foods, as it is difficult to keep wood in a sanitary condition. Uncleanliness of dishes in which foods are placed is too often caused by the use of foul dishcloths and failure to thoroughly wash and rinse the dishes. It is always well to rinse dishes with scalding water, as colds and skin diseases may be communicated from the edges of drinking glasses, and from forks and spoons, and, unless the dish towels are kept scrupulously clean, it is more sanitary to drain the dishes than to wipe them.

286. Contamination from Unclean Dishcloths.--When the dishcloth is foul, the fat absorbed by the fibers becomes rancid, the proteids undergo putrefaction changes with formation of ill-smelling gases containing nitrogen, the carbohydrates ferment and are particularly attractive to flies, and all the various disease germs collected on the surface of the dishcloth are, along with the rancid fat and other putrifying materials, distributed over the surface of the dishes with which the cloth comes in contact.

287. Refrigeration.--At a low temperature the insoluble or unorganized ferments become inactive, but the chemical ferments or enzymes are still capable of carrying on fermentation. Thus it is that a food, when placed in a refrigerator or in cold storage, continues to undergo chemical change. An example of such enzymic action is the curing of beef and cheese in cold storage. A small amount of ventilation is required when foods are refrigerated, just sufficient to keep up a slight circulation of air. It seems not to be generally understood that all fermentation changes do not cease when food is placed in refrigerators, and this often leads to neglect in their care. Cleanliness is equally as essential, or more so, in the refrigeration of food as in its handling in other ways. Too often the refrigerator is neglected, milk and other food is spilt, filling the cracks, and slow decomposition sets in. A well-cared-for refrigerator is an important factor in the preservation of food, but when it is neglected, it becomes a source of contamination. Unclean

vegetables and food receptacles, impure ice and foul air, are the most common forms of contamination. The chemical changes which foods undergo during refrigeration are such as result in softening of the tissues.

288. Soil.--The soil about dwellings and places where foods are stored frequently becomes polluted with decaying animal and vegetable matter, and in such soils disease-producing organisms readily find lodgment. Poorly drained soils containing an excess of vegetable matter furnish a medium in which the tapeworm and the germs of typhoid fever, lockjaw, and various diseases affecting the digestive tract, may propagate. The wind carries the dust particles from these contaminated places into unprotected food, where they cause fermentation changes and the disease germs multiply. In considering the sanitary condition of a locality, the character of the soil is an important factor. Whenever there is reason to suspect that a soil is unsanitary, it should be disinfected with lime or formaldehyde. Soils about dwellings need care and frequent disinfecting to keep them in a sanitary condition, equally as much as do the rooms in the dwellings.[99] In the growing of garden vegetables, frequently large quantities of fertilizers of unsanitary character are used, and vegetables often retain mechanically on their surfaces particles of these. To this dirt clinging to the vegetables have been traced diseases, as typhoid fever and various digestion disorders.

289. Disposal of Kitchen Refuse.--Refuse, as vegetable parings, bones, and meat scraps, unless they are used for food for animals or collected as garbage, should preferably be burned; then there is no danger of their furnishing propagating media for disease germs. Garbage cans should be kept clean, and well covered to protect the contents from flies. Where the refuse cannot be burned, it should be composted. For this, a well-drained place should be selected, and the refuse should be kept covered with earth to keep off the flies and absorb the odors that arise from the fermenting material, and to prevent its being carried away by the wind. Lime should be sprinkled about the compost heap, and from time to time it should be drawn away and the place covered with clean earth. It is very unsanitary to throw all of the kitchen refuse in the same place year after year without resorting to

any means for keeping the soil in a sanitary condition. Although composting refuse is not as sanitary as burning, it is far more sanitary than neglecting to care for it at all, as is too frequently the case.

Ground polluted with kitchen refuse containing large amounts of fatty material and soap becomes diseased, so that the natural fermentation changes fail to take place, and the soil becomes "sewage sick" and gets in such a condition that vegetation will not grow. Failure to properly dispose of kitchen refuse is frequently the cause of the spread of germ diseases, through the dust and flies that are attracted by the material and carry the germs from the refuse pile to food.

Where there is no drainage system, disposal of the liquid refuse is a serious problem. Drain basins and cesspools are often resorted to, and these may become additional sources of contamination. As stated in the chapter on well water, direct communication is frequently established between such places and shallow wells. Where the only place for the disposal of waste water is the surface of the ground, it should be thrown some distance from the house and where it will drain from and not toward the well. The land should be well drained and open to the sunlight. Coarse sand and lime should be sprinkled over it frequently, and occasionally the soil should be removed and replaced with fresh. Sunlight, and disinfection of the soil and good drainage are necessary, in order to keep in a sanitary condition the place where the dish water is thrown.

Poor plumbing is often the cause of contaminated food. The gases which escape from unclean traps may carry with them solid particles of organic matter in various stages of decay. The "house side" of traps always ventilates into the rooms, and hence it is important that they be kept scrupulously clean. Where the drip pipe from the refrigerator drains directly into the sewerage system, there is always danger. Special attention should be given to the care of plumbing near places where foods are stored. Frequently there are leaky joints due to settling of the dwellings or to extreme changes in temperature, and the plumbing should be occasionally inspected by one familiar with the subject.[100]

290. General Considerations.--In order to keep food in the most wholesome condition, special care should be taken that all of its surroundings are sanitary. The air, the dishes in which the food is placed, the refrigerator, cellar or closet where stored, and the other food with which it comes in contact, all influence the wholesomeness or cause contamination. A food may contain sufficient nutrients to give it high value, and yet, on account of products formed during fermentation, be poisonous. Foods are particularly susceptible to putrefaction changes, and chemicals and preservatives added as preventives, with a view of retarding these changes, are objectionable, besides failing to prevent all fermentation from taking place. Intelligent thought should be exercised in the care of food, for the health of the consumer is largely dependent upon the purity and wholesomeness of the food supply.

BY ALLOWING A HOUSE FLY TO CRAWL OVER SURFACE.

(From Minnesota Experiment Station Bulletin No. 93.)]

CHAPTER XXI

LABORATORY PRACTICE

Object of Laboratory Practice, Laboratory Note-book, and Suggestions for Laboratory Practice.--The aim of the laboratory practice is to give the students an idea of the composition, uses, and values of food materials, and the part which chemistry takes in sanitation and household affairs; also to enable them by simple tests to detect some of the more common adulterants in foods.

Before performing an experiment, the student is advised to review those topics presented in the text which have a bearing upon the experiment, so that a clear conception may be gained of the relationship between the laboratory work and that of the class room. The student should endeavor to cultivate the power of observation and to grasp the principle involved in the work, rather than do it in a merely mechanical and perfunctory way. Neatness is one of the essentials for success in laboratory practice, and too much emphasis cannot be laid upon this requisite to good work. The student should learn to use his time in the laboratory profitably and economically. He should obtain a clear idea of what he is to do, and then do it to the best of his ability. If the experiment is not a success, repeat it. While the work is in progress it should be given undivided attention. Care should be exercised to prevent anything getting into the sinks that will clog the plumbing; soil, matches, broken glass, and paper should be deposited in the waste jars.

A careful record of the experiments should be kept by each student in a suitable note-book. It is suggested that those students desiring more time in writing out the experiments than the laboratory period affords, take notes as they make the various tests, and then amplify and rearrange them in the evening study time. The final writing up of the notes should, however, be done before the next laboratory period. Careful attention should be given to the spelling, language, and punctuation, and the note-book should represent the student's individual work. He who attempts to cheat by copying the results of others, only cheats himself. In recording the results of an experiment, the student should state briefly and clearly the following:

1. Number and title of experiment. 2. How the experiment is performed. 3. What was observed. 4. What the experiment proves.

LIST OF APPARATUS USED IN EXPERIMENTS

1 Crucible Tongs 2 Evaporating Dishes 1 Casserole 6 Beakers 12 Test Tubes 1 Wooden Stand 1 Test Tube Stand 1 Sand Bath 2 Funnels 1 Tripod 1 Stoddart Test Tube Clamp 1 Test Tube Brush 1 Burner and Tubing 2 Stirring Rods 6 Watch Glasses 2 Erlenmeyer Flasks 1 Package Filter Paper 1 Box Matches 1 Wire Gauze 2 Burettes 1 Porcelain Crucible 1 Aluminum Dish

Directions for Weighing.--Place the dish or material to be weighed in the left-hand pan of the balance. With the forceps lay a weight from the weight box on the right-hand pan. Do not touch the weights with the hands. If the weight selected is too heavy, replace it with a lighter weight. Add weights until the pans are counterpoised; this will be indicated by the needle swinging nearly as many divisions on one side of the scale as on the other. The brass weights are the gram weights. The other weights are fractions of a gm. The 500, 200, 100 mg. (milligram) weights are recorded as 0.5, 0.2, and 0.1 gm. The 50, 20, and 10 mg. weights as 0.05, 0.02, and 0.01 gm. If the 10, and 2 gm., and the 200, the 100, and the 50 mg. weights are used, the resulting weight is 12.35 gms. No moist substances should ever come in contact with the scale pans. The weights and forceps should always be replaced in the weight box. Too much care and neatness cannot be exercised in weighing.

Directions for Measuring.--Reagents are measured in graduated cylinders (see Fig. 74). When the directions call for the addition of 5 or 10 cc. of a reagent, unless so directed it is not absolutely necessary to measure the reagent in a measuring cylinder. A large test tube holds about 30 cc. of water. Measure out 5 cc. of water and transfer it to a large test tube. Note its volume. Add approximately 5 cc. of water directly to the test tube. Measure it. Repeat this operation until you can judge with a fair degree of accuracy the part of a test tube filled by 5 cc. In the experiments where a burette is used for measuring reagents, the burette is first filled with the reagent by means of a funnel. The tip of the burette is allowed to fill before the readings are made, which are from the lowest point or meniscus. When reagents are removed from bottles, the stopper should be held between the first and second fingers of the right hand (see Fig. 75). Hold the test tube or receptacle that is to receive the reagent in the left hand. Pour the liquid slowly until the desired amount is secured. Before inserting the stopper, touch it to the neck of the bottle to catch the few drops on the edge, thus preventing their streaking down the sides of the bottle on to the shelf. Replace the bottle in its proper place. Every precaution should be taken to prevent contamination of reagents.

1, eye-piece or ocular; 2, objective; 3, stage; 4, cover glass; 5, slide; 6, mirror.]

Use of the Microscope.--Special directions in the use of the microscope will be given by the instructor. The object or material to be examined is placed on a microscopical slide. Care should be exercised to secure a representative sample, and to properly distribute the substance on the slide. If a pulverized material is to be examined, use but little and spread it in as thin a layer as possible. If a liquid, one or two drops placed on the slide will suffice. The material on the slide is covered with a cover glass, before it is placed on the stage of the microscope. In focusing, do not allow the object glass of the microscope to come in contact with the cover glass. Focus upward, not downward. Special care should be exercised in focusing and in handling the eye-piece and objective. A camel's-hair brush, clean dry chamois skin, or clean silk only should be used in polishing the lenses. Always put the microscope back in its case after using.

Experiment No. 1

Water in Flour

Carefully weigh a porcelain or aluminum dish. (Porcelain must be used if the ash is to be determined on the same sample.) Place in it about 2 gm. of flour; record the weight; then place the dish in the water oven for at least 6 hours. After drying, weigh again, and from the loss of weight calculate the per cent of water in the flour. (Weight of flour and dish before drying minus weight of flour and dish after drying equals weight of water lost. Weight of water divided by weight of flour taken, multiplied by 100, equals the per cent of water in the flour.)

How does the amount of water you obtained compare with the amount given in the tables of analysis?

Experiment No. 2

Water in Butter

Carefully weigh a clean, dry aluminum dish, place in it about 2 gms. of butter, and weigh again. Record the weights. Place the dish containing butter in the water oven for 5 or 6 hours and then weigh. The loss in weight represents the water in the butter. Calculate the per cent of water. Care must be taken to get a representative sample of the butter to be tested; preferably small amounts should be taken with the butter trier from various parts of the package.

Experiment No. 3

Ash in Flour

Place the porcelain dish containing flour from the preceding experiment in a muffle furnace and let it remain until the organic matter is completely volatilized. Cool, weigh, and determine the per cent of ash. The flour should be burned at the lowest temperature necessary for complete combustion.

Experiment No. 4

Nitric Acid Test for Nitrogenous Organic Matter

To 3 cc. of egg albumin in a test tube add 2 cc. of HNO_3 (conc.) and heat. When cool add NH_4OH. The nitric acid chemically reacts upon the albumin, forming yellow xanthoprotein. What change occurs in the appearance of the egg albumin when the HNO_3 is added? Is this a physical or chemical change? What is the name of the compound formed? What change occurs on adding NH_4OH?

Experiment No. 5

Acidity of Lemons

With a pipette measure into a small beaker 2 cc. of lemon juice. Add 25 cc. of water and a few drops of phenolphthalein indicator. From the burette run in N/10 KOH solution until a faint pink tinge remains permanently. Note the number of cubic centimeters of KOH solution required to neutralize the citric acid in the lemon juice. Calculate the per cent of citric acid.

(1 cc. of N/10 KOH solution equals 0.00642 gm. citric acid. 1 cc. of H_2O weighs 1 gm. Because of sugar and other matter in solution 1 cc. of lemon juice weighs approximately 1.03 gm.)

1. What is the characteristic acid of lemons? 2. What is the salt formed when the lemon juice is neutralized by the KOH solution? 3. Describe briefly the process for determining the acidity of lemon juice. 4. What per cent of acidity did you obtain? 5. How does this compare with the acidity of vinegar?

Experiment No. 6

Influence of Heat on Potato Starch Grains

With the point of a knife scrape slightly the surface of a raw potato and place a drop of the starchy juice upon the microscopical slide. Cover with cover glass and examine under the microscope.

In the evaporating dish cook a small piece of potato, then place a very small portion upon the slide, and examine with the microscope.

Make drawings of the starch grains in raw and in cooked potatoes.

Experiment No. 7

Influence of Yeast on Starch Grains

Moisten a small portion of the dough prepared with yeast and with the stirring rod place a drop of the starchy water upon the slide. Cover with cover glass and examine under the microscope.

Repeat, examining a drop of starchy water washed from flour.

Make drawing of wheat starch grain in flour and in dough prepared with yeast.

Experiment No. 8

Mechanical Composition of Potatoes

Wash one potato. Weigh, then peel, making the peeling as thin as possible. Weigh the peeled potato and weigh the peeling or refuse. Calculate the per cent of potato that is edible and the per cent that is refuse.

Experiment No. 9

Pectose from Apples

Reduce a small peeled apple to a pulp. Squeeze the pulp through a clean cloth into a beaker. Add 10 cc. H_2O and heat on a sand bath to coagulate the albumin. Filter, adding a little hot water if necessary. To the filtrate add 5 cc. alcohol. The precipitate is the pectose material.

1. Is the pectose from the apple soluble? 2. Is it coagulated by heat? 3. Is it soluble in alcohol?

Experiment No. 10

Lemon Extract

To 5 cc. of the extract in a test tube add an equal volume of water. A cloudy appearance indicates the presence of lemon oil. If the solution remains clear after adding the water, the extract does not contain lemon oil.

Why does the extract containing lemon oil become cloudy on adding water?

Experiment No. 11

Vanilla Extract

Pour into a test tube 5 cc. of the extract to be tested. Evaporate to one third. Then add sufficient water to restore the original volume. If a brown, flocculent precipitate is formed, the sample contains pure vanilla extract. Resin is present in vanilla beans and is extracted in the essence. The resin is readily soluble in 50 per cent alcohol. If the alcohol is removed from the extract, the excess of resin is precipitated, or if free from alkali, it may be precipitated by diluting the original solution with twice its volume of water. Test the two samples and compare.

(Adapted from Leach, "Food Inspection and Analysis.")

1. Describe the appearance of each sample after evaporating and adding water. 2. Which sample contains pure vanilla extract? 3. State the principle underlying this test.

Experiment No. 12

Testing Olive Oil for Cotton Seed Oil

Pour into a test tube 5 cc. of the oil to be tested and 5 cc. of Halphen's Reagent. Mix thoroughly. Plug the test tube loosely with cotton, and heat in a bath of boiling saturated brine for 15 minutes. If cotton seed oil is present, a deep red or orange color is produced. Test two samples and compare.

Halphen's Reagent.--Mix equal volumes of amyl alcohol and carbon disulphid containing about one per cent of sulphur in solution.

(Adapted from Leach, "Food Inspection and Analysis.")

Experiment No. 13

Testing for Coal Tar Dyes

Dilute 20 to 30 cc. of the material to 100 cc.; boil for 10 minutes with 10 cc. of a 10 per cent solution of potassium bisulphate and a piece of white woolen cloth which has previously been boiled in a 0.1 per cent solution of NaOH and thoroughly washed in water. Remove the cloth from the solution, wash in boiling water, and dry between pieces of filter paper. A bright red indicates coal tar dye. If the coloring matter is entirely from fruit, the woolen cloth will be either uncolored or will have a faint pink or brown color which is changed to green or yellow by ammonia and is not restored by washing. This is the Arata test.

(Adapted, Winston, Conn. Experiment Station Report.)

1. Describe Arata's wool test for coal tar dyes. 2. What is the appearance of the woolen cloth when the coloring matter is entirely from fruit? 3. What effect has NH_4OH upon the color? 4. Why is NaOH used? 5. Why may not cotton cloth be used instead of woolen? 6. What can you say of the use of coal tar dyes in foods?

Experiment No. 14

Determining the Per Cent of Skin in Beans

Place in an evaporating dish 10 gm. of beans, 50 cc. of water, and 1/2 gm. of baking soda. Boil 10 minutes or until the skins are loosened, then drain off the water. Add cold water and rub the beans together till the skins slip off. Collect the skins, place on a watch glass and dry in the water oven for 1/2 hour. Weigh the dried skins and calculate the per cent of "skin."

1. What does the soda do? 2. What effect would hard limewater have upon the skins? 3. How does removal of skins affect food value of beans and digestibility?

Experiment No. 15

Extraction of Fat from Peanuts

Shell three or four peanuts and with the mortar and pestle break them into small pieces. Place in a test tube and pour over them about 10 cc. of ether. Cork the test tube and allow it to stand 30 minutes, shaking occasionally. Filter on to a watch glass and let stand until the ether evaporates, and then observe the fat.

1. What is the appearance of the peanut fat? 2. What is the solvent of the fat? 3. What becomes of the ether? 4. Why should the peanuts be broken into small pieces?

Experiment No. 16

Microscopic Examination of Milk

Place a drop of milk on a microscopical slide and cover with cover glass. Examine the milk to detect impurities, as dust, hair, refuse, etc. Make drawings of any foreign matter present.

Experiment No. 17

Formaldehyde in Cream or Milk

To 10 cc. of milk in a casserole add 10 cc. of the acid reagent. Heat slowly over the flame nearly to boiling, holding the casserole in the hand and giving it a slight rotary movement while heating. The presence of formaldehyde is indicated by a violet coloration varying in depth with the amount present. In the absence of formaldehyde the solution slowly turns brown.

Acid Reagent.--Commercial hydrochloric acid (sp. gr. 1.2) containing 2 cc. per liter of 10 per cent ferric chlorid.

(Adapted from Leach, "Food Inspection and Analysis.")

1. How may the presence of formaldehyde in milk be detected? 2. Why in this test is it necessary to use acid containing ferric chlorid? 3. Describe the appearance of the two samples of milk after adding the acid reagent and heating. 4. Which sample showed the presence of formaldehyde?

Experiment No. 18

Gelatine in Cream or Milk

To 20 cc. of milk or cream in a beaker add 20 cc. of acid mercuric nitrate and about 40 cc. of H_2O. Let stand for a few minutes and filter. Filtrate will be cloudy if gelatine is present.

Add 1/2 cc. of a dilute solution of picric acid--a heavy yellow precipitate indicates gelatine.

Acid Mercuric Nitrate.--1 part by weight of Hg, 2 parts HNO_3 (sp. gr. 1.42). Dilute 25 times with water.

Experiment No. 19

Testing for Oleomargarine

Apply the following tests to two samples of the material:

Boiling or Spoon Test.--Melt the sample to be tested--a piece about the size of a chestnut--in a large spoon, hastening the process by stirring with a splinter. Then, increasing the heat, bring to as brisk a boil as possible and stir thoroughly, not neglecting the outer edges. Oleomargarine and renovated butter boil noisily, sputtering like a mixture of grease and water, and produce no foam, or but very little. Genuine butter boils with less noise and produces an abundance of foam.

Waterhouse Test.--Into a small beaker pour 50 cc. of sweet milk. Heat nearly to boiling and add from 5 to 10 gms. of butter or oleomargarine. Stir with a glass rod until fat is melted. Then place the beaker in cold water and stir the milk until the temperature falls sufficiently for the fat to congeal. At this point the fat, if oleomargarine, can easily be collected into one lump by means of the rod; while if butter, it will granulate and cannot be collected.

(From Farmers' Bul. 131, U. S. Dept. of Agriculture.)

1. Name two simple tests for distinguishing butter and oleomargarine. 2. Describe these tests. 3. Why do butter and oleomargarine respond differently to these tests? 4. Are these tests based upon chemical or physical properties of the fats?

Experiment No. 20

Testing for Watering or Skimming of Milk

a. Fat Content of Milk by Means of Babcock Test.--Measure with pipette into test bottle 17.6 cc. of milk. Sample should be carefully taken and well mixed. Measure with cylinder 17.5 cc. commercial H_2SO_4 and add to milk in test bottle. (See Fig. 25.) Mix acid and milk by rotating the bottle. Then place test bottles in centrifugal machine and whirl 5 minutes. Add sufficient hot water to test bottles to bring contents up to about the 8th mark on stem. Then whirl bottles 2 minutes longer and read fat. Read from extreme lowest to highest point. Each large division as 1 to 2 represents a whole per cent, each small division 0.2 of a per cent.

b. Determining Specific Gravity by Means of Lactometer.--Pour 150 cc. of milk into 200 cc. cylinder. Place lactometer in milk and note depth to which it sinks as indicated on stem. Note also temperature of milk. For each 10?above 60?F. add 1 to the lactometer number, in order to make the necessary correction for temperature. For example, if milk has sp. gr. of 1.032 at temperature of 70? it will be equivalent to sp. gr. of 1.033 at 60? Ordinarily milk has a sp. gr. of 1.029 to 1.034. If milk has sp. gr. less than 1.029, or contains less than 3 per cent fat, it may be considered watered milk. If the milk has a high sp. gr. (above 1.035) and a low content of fat, some of the fat has been removed.

(For extended direction for milk testing see Snyder's "Dairy Chemistry.")

Experiment No. 21

Boric Acid in Meat

Cut into very small pieces 5 gms, of meat, removing all the fat possible. Place in an evaporating dish with 20 to 25 cc. of water to which a few drops of HCl have been added and warm slightly. Dip a piece of turmeric paper in the meat extract and dry. A rose-red color of the turmeric paper after drying (turned olive by a weak ammonia solution) is indicative of boric acid.

1. How may meat be tested for boric acid? 2. Why is HCl added to the water? 3. Why is the water containing the meat warmed slightly? 4. What is the appearance of the turmeric paper after being dipped in the meat extract and dried? 5. What change takes place when it is moistened with ammonia, and why?

Experiment No. 22

Microscopic Examination of Cereal Starch Grains

Make a microscopic examination and drawings of wheat, corn, rice, and oat starch grains, comparing them with the drawings of the different starch grains on the chart. If the material is coarse, pulverize in a mortar and filter through cloth. Place a drop or two of the starchy water on the slide, cover with a cover glass, and examine.

Experiment No. 23

Identification of Commercial Cereals

Examine under the microscope two samples of cereal breakfast foods, and by comparison with the wheat, corn, and oat starch grains previously examined tell of what grains the breakfast foods are made and their approximate food value.

Experiment No. 24

Granulation and Color of Flour

Arrange on glass plate, in order of color, samples of all the different grades of flour. Note the differences in color. How do these differences correspond with the grades of the flour? Examine the flour with a microscope, noting any coarse or dark-colored particles of bran or dust. Rub some of the flour between the thumb and forefinger. Note if any granular particles can be detected.

Experiment No. 25

Capacity of Flour to absorb Water

Weigh out 15 gms. of soft wheat flour into an evaporating dish; then add from burette a measured quantity of water sufficient to make a stiff dough. Note the amount of water required for this purpose. Repeat the operation, using hard wheat flour.

1. How may the absorptive power of a flour be determined? 2. To what is it due? 3. Why do some flours absorb more water than others?

Experiment No. 26

Acidity of Flour

Weigh into a flask 20 gms. of flour and add 200 cc. distilled water. Shake vigorously. After letting stand 30 minutes, filter and then titrate 50 cc. of the filtrate against standard KOH solution, using phenolphthalein as indicator, 1 cc. of the alkali equals 0.009 gms. lactic acid. Calculate the per cent of acid present.

1. How may the acidity of a flour be determined? 2. The acidity is expressed in percentage amounts of what acid? 3. What per cent of acidity is found in normal flours? 4. What does a high acidity of a flour indicate?

Experiment No. 27

Moist and Dry Gluten

Weigh 30 gms. of flour into a porcelain dish. Make the flour into a stiff dough. After 30 minutes obtain the gluten by washing, being careful to remove all the starch and prevent any losses. Squeeze the water from the gluten as thoroughly as possible. Weigh the moist gluten and calculate the per cent. Dry the gluten in the water oven and calculate the per cent of dry gluten.

Experiment No. 28

Gliadin from Flour

Place in a flask 10 gms. of flour, 30 cc. of alcohol, and 20 cc. of water. Cork the flask and shake, and after a few minutes shake again. Allow the alcohol to act on the flour for an hour, or until the next day. Then filter off the alcohol solution and evaporate the filtrate to dryness over the water bath. Examine the residue; to a portion add a little water; burn a small portion and observe odor.

1. Describe the appearance of the gliadin. 2. What was the result when water was added? 3. When burned, what was the odor of the gliadin, and what does this indicate? 4. What is gliadin?

Experiment No. 29

Bread-making Test

Make a "sponge" by mixing together:

12 gm. sugar, 12 gm. yeast (compressed), 4 gm. salt, 175 cc. water (temp. 32?C.).

Let stand 1/2 hour at a temperature of 30?C. In a large bowl, mix with a knife or spatula 7.7 gms. of lard with 248.6 gms. of flour. Then add 160 cc. of the "sponge," or as much as is needed to make a good stiff dough, and mix thoroughly, using the spatula. With some flours as small a quantity as 150 cc. of sponge may be used. If more moisture is necessary, add H_2O. Keep at temperature of 30?C. Allow the dough to stand 50 minutes to first pulling, 40 minutes to second pulling, and 30 to 50 minutes to the pan. Let it rise to top of pan and then bake for 1/2 hour in an oven at a temperature of 180?C. One loaf of bread is made of patent flour of known quality as a standard for comparison, and other loaves of the flours to be tested. Compare the loaves as to size (cubic contents), color, porosity, odor, taste, nature of crust, and form of loaf.

Experiment No. 30

Microscopic Examination of Yeast

On a watch glass mix thoroughly a very small piece of yeast with about 5 cc. of water and then with the stirring rod place a drop of this solution on the microscopical slide, adding a drop of very dilute methyl violet solution. Cover with the cover glass and examine under the microscope. The living active cells appear colorless while the decayed and lifeless ones are stained. Yeast cells are circular or oval in shape. (See Fig. 46.)

(Adapted from Leach, "Food Inspection and Analysis.")

Experiment No. 31

Testing Baking Powders for Alum

Place about 2 gms. of flour in a dish with 1/2 gm. baking powder. Add enough water to make a dough and then 2 or 3 drops of tincture of logwood and 2 or 3 drops of ammonium carbonate solution. Mix well and observe; a blue color indicates alum. Try the same test, using flour only for comparison.

1. How do you test a baking powder for alum? 2. What difference in color did you observe in the test with the baking powder containing alum and in that with the flour only? 3. Why is the $(NH_4)_2CO_3$ solution used?

Experiment No. 32

Testing Baking Powders for Phosphoric Acid

Dissolve 1/2 gm. of baking powder in 5 cc. of H_2O and 3 cc. HNO_3. Filter and add 3 cc. ammonium molybdate. Heat gently. A yellow precipitate indicates phosphoric acid.

1. How do you test a baking powder for phosphoric acid? 2. What is the yellow precipitate obtained in this test?

Experiment No. 33

Testing Baking Powders for Ammonia

Dissolve 1/2 gm. of material in 10 cc. water; filter off any insoluble residue and to the filtrate add 2 or 3 cc. NaOH and apply heat. Test the gas given off with moistened turmeric paper. If NH_3 is present, the paper will be colored brown. Do not allow the paper to come in contact with the liquid or sides of the test tube. (Perform the tests on two samples of baking powder.)

1. How do you test a baking powder for ammonia? 2. Why do you add NaOH? 3. Why must you be careful not to let the turmeric paper touch the sides of the test tube or the liquid?

Experiment No. 34

Vinegar Solids

Into a weighed aluminum or porcelain dish pour 10 cc. of vinegar. Weigh and then evaporate over boiling water. To drive off the last traces of moisture dry in the water oven for an hour. Cool and weigh. Calculate the per cent of solids. Observe the appearance of the solids. Test both samples and compare.

1. How may the per cent of solids in vinegar be determined? 2. Describe the appearance of the solids from the good and from the poor sample of vinegar. 3. What is the legal standard for vinegar solids in your state?

Experiment No. 35

Specific Gravity of Vinegar

Pour 170 cc. vinegar into 200 cc. cylinder. Place a hydrometer for heavy liquids (sp. gr. 1 to 1.1) in the cylinder. Note the depth to which it sinks and the point registered on the scale on the stem. Note temperature of vinegar. Record specific gravity of vinegar.

1. What effect would addition of water to vinegar have upon its specific gravity? 2. What effect would addition of such material as sugar have upon specific gravity? 3. Why should the specific gravity of vinegar be fairly constant? 4. What would be the weight of 1000 cc. of vinegar calculated from the specific gravity?

Experiment No. 36

Acidity of Vinegar

Into a small beaker pour 6 cc. of vinegar and 10 cc. of water and a few drops of phenolphthalein indicator. Run in standard KOH solution from a burette until a faint pink tinge remains permanently. Note the number of cubic centimeters of KOH solution required to neutralize the acid. Divide this number by 10, which will give approximately the per cent of acetic acid.

1. How may the per cent of acidity of vinegar be determined? 2. Why was phenolphthalein used? 3. Why was KOH used? 4. What acids does vinegar contain? 5. What is the legal requirement in this state for acetic acid in vinegar? 6. How did the acidity you obtained compare with this legal requirement?

Experiment No. 37

Deportment of Vinegar with Reagents

To 10 cc. of vinegar in a test tube add 8 or 10 drops of lead sub-acetate and shake. Observe the precipitate. Lead sub-acetate precipitates mainly the malic acid which is always present in cider vinegar.

1. How may the presence of malic acid in a vinegar be detected? 2. Describe the precipitate. 3. What does malic acid in a vinegar indicate?

Experiment No. 38

Testing Mustard for Turmeric

Place 1 gm. of ground mustard on a small watch glass and moisten slightly with water. Add 2 or 3 drops of NH_4OH, stirring well with a glass rod. A brown color indicates turmeric present in considerable quantity.

Test a sample of good mustard and one adulterated with turmeric and compare the results.

Experiment No. 39

Examination of Tea Leaves

Soak a small amount of tea and unroll 8 or 10 of the leaves. Make a drawing of a tea leaf. Observe the proportion of stems in each of three samples of tea; also the relative proportion of large and small leaves. Observe if the leaves are even as to size and of a uniform color.

Experiment No. 40

Action of Iron Compounds upon Tannic Acid

Make an infusion of tea by placing 3 gms. of tea in 100 cc. of hot water and stirring well. Filter off some of the infusion and test 5 cc. with ferrous sulphate solution made by dissolving 1 gm. $FeSO_4$ in 10 cc. H_2O and filtering. Note the result.

1. What change in color did you observe when the ferrous sulphate solution was added to the tea infusion? 2. What effect would waters containing iron have upon the tea infusion?

Experiment No. 41

Identification of Coffee Berries

Examine Rio, Java, and Mocha coffee berries. Describe each. Note the characteristics of each kind of coffee berry.

Experiment No. 42

Detecting Chicory in Coffee

Fill a beaker with water and place about a teaspoonful of ground coffee on the surface. If much of the ground material sinks and it imparts a dark brown color to the lower portion of the liquid, it is an indication of the presence of chicory. Pure coffee floats on water. Chicory has a higher specific gravity than coffee.

1. How may the presence of chicory in ground coffee be detected? 2. Why does coffee float on the water while chicory sinks? 3. What effect does chicory have upon the color of water?

Experiment No. 43

Testing Hard and Soft Waters

Partially fill a large cylinder with very hard water. This may be prepared by dissolving 0.1 to 0.2 gm. calcium chloride in 500 cc. of ordinary water. Add to this a measured quantity of soap solution. Mix well and notice how many cubic centimeters of soap solution must be used before a permanent lather is formed, also notice the precipitate of "lime soap." Repeat this experiment, using either rain or distilled water, and compare the cubic centimeters of soap solution used with that in former test. Repeat the test, using tap water.

Soap Solution.--Scrape 10 gms. of castile soap into fine shavings and dissolve in a liter of alcohol, dilute with 1/3 water. Filter if not clear and keep in a tightly stoppered bottle.

1. Why is more soap required to form a lather with hard water than with soft water? 2. What is meant by "lime soap"? Describe its appearance. 3. How may hard waters be softened for household purposes?

Experiment No. 44

Solvent Action of Water on Lead

Put 1 gm. of clean bright lead shavings into a test tube containing 10 cc. of distilled water. After 24 hours decant the clear liquid into a second test tube, acidify slightly with HCL, and add a little hydrogen sulphid water. A black or brownish coloration indicates lead in solution.

(Adapted from Caldwell and Breneman, "Introductory Chemical Practice.")

Under what conditions may lead pipes be objectionable?

Experiment No. 45

Suspended Matter in Water

Place a drop of water on the microscopical slide, cover with cover glass, and examine with the microscope. Note the occurrence and appearance of any suspended matter in the water.

Experiment No. 46

Organic Matter in Water

Pour into the evaporating dish 100 cc. H_2O and evaporate to dryness over the sand bath. Ignite the solids. If the solids blacken when ignited, the water contains organic matter.

Experiment No. 47

Deposition of Lime by Boiling Water

Boil for a few minutes about 200 cc. of water in a flask. After the water is cool, note any sediment of lime or turbidity of the water due to expelling the carbon dioxid.

1. What is meant by a "hard" water? 2. What do the terms "temporary" and "permanent" hardness of water mean? 3. What acts as a solvent of the lime in water? 4. Why does boiling cause the lime to be deposited?

Experiment No. 48

Qualitative Tests for Minerals in Water

Test for Chlorids.--To 10 cc. of H_2O add a few drops of HNO_3 and 2 cc. of $AgNO_3$. A white precipitate indicates the presence of chlorids, usually in the form of sodium chlorid.

Test for Sulphates.--To 10 cc. of water add 2 cc. of dilute HCl and 2 cc. of $BaCl_2$. A cloudiness or the formation of a white precipitate indicates the presence of sulphates.

Test for Iron.--If a brown sediment is formed in water exposed to the air for some time, it is probably iron hydroxid. To 10 cc. of the water add a few drops of HNO_3, heat, and then add 1/2 cc. of NH_4CNS. A red color indicates the presence of iron.

Test for CaO and MgO.--To 10 cc. of H_2O add 5 cc. NH_4OH. If a precipitate forms, filter it off, and to the filtrate add 3 cc. NH_4Cl and 5 cc. $(NH_4)_2C_2O_4$. The precipitate is CaC_2O_4, and the filtrate contains the magnesia. Filter and add 5 cc. Na_3PO_4 to precipitate $MgNH_4PO_4$.

1. How would you test a water to detect the presence of organic matter? 2. Name some mineral impurities often found in water. 3. Describe the test for chlorids; for sulphates; for iron; for lime; for magnesium. 4. Of the two classes of impurities found in water, which is the more harmful? 5. Name three ways of purifying waters known to be impure, and tell which is the most effectual.

Experiment No. 49

Testing for Nitrites in Water

To 50 cc. of water in a small beaker add with a pipette 2 cc. of naphthylamine hydrochloride and then 2 cc. of sulphanilic acid. Stir well and wait 20 minutes for color to develop. A pink color indicates nitrites.

REAGENTS USED

Sulphanilic Acid.--Dissolve 5 gm. in 150 cc. of dilute acetic acid; sp. gr. 1.04.

Naphthylamine Hydrochloride.--Boil 0.1 gm. of solid [Greek: a]-amidonaphthaline (naphthylamine) in 20 cc. of water, filter the solution through a plug of absorbent cotton, and mix the nitrate with 180 cc. of dilute acetic acid. All water used must be free from nitrites, and all vessels must be rinsed out with such water before tests are applied.

1. Would a water showing the presence of nitrites be a safe drinking water? Why? 2. What are nitrites? 3. What does the presence of nitrites indicate? 4. Are small amounts of nitrites, when not associated with bacteria, injurious?

REVIEW QUESTIONS

CHAPTER I

GENERAL COMPOSITION OF FOODS

1. To what extent is water present in foods? 2. What foods contain the most, and what foods the least water? 3. How does the water content of some foods vary with the hydroscopicity of the air? 4. How may changes in water content of foods affect their weight? 5. Why is it necessary to consider the water content of foods in assigning nutritive values? 6. How is the dry matter of a food determined? 7. Why is the determination of the water in a food often a difficult process? 8. What is the ash or mineral matter of a food? 9. How is it obtained? 10. What is its source? 11. Of what is the ash of plants composed? 12. What part in plant life do these ash elements take? 13. Name the ash elements essential for plant growth. 14. Which of the mineral elements take the most essential part in animal nutrition? 15. In what form are these elements usually considered most valuable? 16. Why is sodium chloride or common salt necessary for animal life? 17. How do food materials differ in ash content? 18. Define organic matter of foods. 19. How is it obtained? 20. Of what is it composed? 21. Into what is the organic matter converted when it is burned? 22. Give the two large classes of organic compounds found in food materials. 23. Name the various subdivisions of the non-nitrogenous compounds. 24. What are the carbohydrates? 25. Give their general composition. 26. What is cellulose? 27. Where is it found? 28. What is its function in plants? 29. What is its food value? 30. In what way may cellulose be of value in a ration? 31. In what way may it impart a negative value to a ration? 32. What is starch? 33. Where is it mainly found in plants? 34. Give the mechanical structure of the starch grain. 35. Why is starch insoluble in cold water? 36. How do starch

grains from different sources differ in structure? 37. What effect does heat have upon starch? 38. Define hydration of starch. 39. Under what conditions does this change take place? 40. What value as a nutrient does starch possess? 41. What is sugar? 42. How does it resemble and how differ in composition from starch? 43. What are the pectose substances? 44. How are they affected by heat? 45. What food value do they possess? 46. What is nitrogen-free-extract? 47. How is it obtained? 48. How may the nitrogen-free-extract of one food differ from that of another? 49. What are the fats? 50. How do they differ in composition from the starches? 51. Why does fat when burned or digested produce more heat than starch or sugar? 52. Name the separate fats of which animal and vegetable foods are composed. 53. Give some of the physical characteristics of fat. 54. What is the iodine absorption number of a fat? 55. How does the specific gravity of fat compare with that of water? 56. Into what two constituents may all fats be separated? 57. What is ether extract? 58. How does the ether extract in fats vary in composition and nutritive value? 59. What are the organic acids? 60. Name those most commonly met with in foods. 61. What nutritive value do they possess? 62. What dietetic value? 63. What value are they to the growing plant? 64. What organic acids are found in animal foods? 65. What are the essential oils? 66. How do they differ from the fixed oils, or fats? 67. What property do the essential oils impart to foods? 68. What food value do they possess? 69. What dietetic value? 70. What are the mixed compounds? 71. How may a compound impart a negative value to a food? 72. What is the nutritive value of the non-nitrogenous compounds, taken as a class? 73. Why is it necessary that nitrogenous and non-nitrogenous compounds be blended in a ration? 74. What are the nitrogenous compounds? 75. How do they differ from the non-nitrogenous compounds? 76. Name the four subdivisions of the nitrogenous compounds. 77. What is protein? 78. What is characteristic as to its nitrogen content? 79. What are some of the derivative products that can be obtained from the protein molecule? 80. How does the protein content of animal bodies compare with that of plants? 81. Name the various subdivisions of the proteins. 82. What is albumin, and how may it be obtained from a food? 83. What is globulin, and how is it obtained from a food? 84. Give some examples of globulins. 85. What are the albuminates, and how are they affected by the action of acids and alkalies? 86. What are the peptones, and how do they differ from the albumins? 87. How are the peptones produced from other proteids? 88. What are the insoluble proteids? 89. Give an example. 90. Which of the proteids are found to the greatest extent in foods? 91. Why may proteids from different sources vary in their nutritive value? 92. What general change do the proteids undergo during digestion? 93. What is crude protein? 94. How is the crude protein content of a food calculated? 95. Why is the nitrogen content of a food more absolute than the crude protein content? 96. What food value do the proteins possess? 97. Why may proteins serve so many functions in the body? 98. Why is protein necessary as a nutrient? 99. What is the effect of an excess of protein in the ration? 100. What is the effect of a scant amount of protein in a ration? 101. What are the albuminoids? 102. Name borne materials that contain large amounts of albuminoids. 103. What food value do the albuminoids possess? 104. What are the amids? 105. How are they formed in plants? 106. What is their source in animals? 107. What general changes does the element nitrogen undergo in plant and animal bodies? 108. What is the food value of the amids? 109. What are the alkaloids? 110. What is their food value? 111. What effect do some alkaloids exert upon the animal body? 112. How may they be produced in animal foods? 113. What general relationship exists between the various nitrogenous compounds? 114. Why is it essential that the animal body be supplied with nitrogenous food in the form of proteids? 115. Name the cycle of changes through which the element nitrogen passes in plant and animal bodies.

CHAPTER II

CHANGES IN COMPOSITION OF FOODS DURING COOKING AND PREPARATION

116. How do raw and cooked foods compare in general composition? 117. In what ways are foods acted upon during cooking? 118. What causes chemical changes to take place during cooking? 119. What are the principal compounds that are changed during the process of cooking? 120. How does

cooking affect the cellulose of foods? 121. What change does starch undergo during cooking? 122. When foods containing starch are baked, what change occurs? 123. How are the sugars acted upon when foods are cooked? 124. What effect does dry heat have upon sugar? 125. What change occurs to the fats during cooking? 126. How does this affect nutritive value? 127. What changes do the proteids undergo during cooking? 128. Why does the action of heat affect various proteids in different ways? 129. Why are chemical changes, as hydration, often desirable in the cooking and preparation of foods? 130. What physical changes do vegetable and animal tissues undergo when cooked? 131. How do foods change in weight during cooking? 132. Why is a prolonged high temperature unnecessary to secure the best results in cooking? 133. To what extent is the energy of fuels utilized for producing mechanical and chemical changes in foods during cooking? 134. What effect does cooking have upon the bacterial flora of foods? 135. In what ways do bacteria exert a favorable influence in the preparation of foods? 136. How may certain classes of bacteria exert unfavorable changes in the preparation of foods? 137. What are the insoluble ferments? 138. What are the soluble ferments? 139. What part do they take in animal and plant nutrition? 140. Define aerobic ferments. 141. Define anabolic ferments. 142. What general relationship exists between the chemical, physical, and bacteriological changes that take place in foods? 143. Why should foods also possess an esthetic value? 144. What kinds of colors should be used in the preparation of foods? 145. What processes should be used for removal of coloring materials from foods?

CHAPTER III

VEGETABLE FOODS

146. Give the general composition of vegetable foods as a class. 147. How do vegetable foods differ from animal foods? 148. Name some vegetables which contain the maximum, and some which contain the minimum percentage of protein. 149. Give the general composition of potatoes. 150. Of what is the dry matter mainly composed? 151. How much of the crude

protein of potatoes is true protein? 152. What ratio exists between the nitrogenous and non-nitrogenous compounds in the potato? 153. Give the chemical composition of the potato. 154. What influence do different methods of boiling have upon the crude protein content of potatoes? 155. To what extent are the nutrients of potatoes digested and absorbed by the body? 156. What value do potatoes impart to the ration? 157. How do sweet potatoes differ in chemical composition and food value from white potatoes? 158. How do carrots differ in composition from potatoes? 159. What is characteristic of the dry matter of the carrot? 160. How do carrots and milk differ in composition? 161. To what is the color of the carrot due? 162. To what extent are the nutrients removed in the cooking of carrots? 163. What is the value of carrots in a ration? 164. Give the characteristics of the composition of parsnips. 165. How does the starch of parsnips differ from that of potatoes? 166. How does the mineral matter of parsnips differ from that of potatoes? 167. How does the cabbage differ in general composition from many vegetables? 168. To what extent are nutrients extracted in the boiling of cabbage? 169. Give the nutritive value of cabbage. 170. How does the cauliflower differ from cabbage? 171. Give the general composition of beets. 172. Give the general composition of cucumbers. 173. What nutritive value has lettuce? 174. Give the composition and dietetic value of onions. 175. How does the ratio of nitrogenous and non-nitrogenous compounds in spinach differ from that in many other vegetables? 176. Give the general composition and nutritive value of asparagus. 177. How much nutritive material do melons contain? 178. What are the principal compounds of tomatoes? 179. What nutrients do they supply to the ration? 180. In the canning of tomatoes, why is it desirable to conserve the juices? 181. How does sweet corn differ in composition from fully matured corn? 182. What nutritive value does the egg plant possess? 183. What are the principal nutrients of squash? 184. What nutritive material does celery contain? 185. To what does celery owe its dietetic value? 186. Why are vegetables necessary in a ration? 187. Why is it not possible to value many vegetable foods simply on the basis of percentage of nutrients present? 188. Name the miscellaneous compounds which many vegetables contain, and the characteristics which these may impart. 189. Why is it necessary to consider the sanitary conditions of vegetables? 190. How do canned vegetables differ in composition and food value from fresh vegetables? 191. What proportion of vegetables is refuse and non-edible parts? 192. Why is it necessary to consider the refuse of a food in determining its nutritive value?

CHAPTER IV

FRUITS

193. To what extent do fruits contain water and dry matter? 194. Give the general composition of fruits. 195. What compounds impart taste and flavor? 196. How much nutrients do fruits add to a ration? 197. Why is it not right to determine the value of fruits entirely on the basis of nutrients? 198. Give the general composition of apples? 199. What compound is present to the greatest extent in the dry matter of apples? 200. How do apples differ in composition? 201. Give the general physical composition of oranges. 202. What nutrients are present to the greatest extent in oranges? 203. How do lemons differ in composition from oranges? 204. How does grape fruit resemble and how differ in chemical composition from oranges and lemons? 205. What are the main compounds in strawberries? 206. In what ways are strawberries valuable in a ration? 207. Of what is grape juice mainly composed? 208. What acid is in grapes, and what is its commercial value? 209. To what are the differences in flavor and taste due? 210. How do ripe olives differ in composition from green olives? 211. What is the food value of the olive? 212. What physiological property does olive oil have? 213. What is the principal nutrient in peaches? 214. What compounds give flavor to peaches? 215. Of what does the dry matter of plums mainly consist? 216. How do plums differ in composition from many other fruits? 217. What are prunes? What is their food value? 218. How do dried fruits differ in composition from fresh fruits? 219. What should be the stage of ripeness of fruit in order to secure the best results in canning? 220. How do canned fruits differ in composition and nutritive value from fresh fruits? 221. To what extent are metals dissolved by fruit juices? 222. Why should tin in which canned goods are preserved be of good quality? 223. What

preservatives are sometimes used in the preparation of canned fruits? 224. What is the objection to their use? 225. Why are fruits necessary in the ration? 226. What change does heat bring about in the pectose substances of fruits?

CHAPTER V

SUGAR, MOLASSES, SIRUPS, HONEY, AND CONFECTIONS

227. What is sugar? 228. From what sources are sugars obtained? 229. Name the two divisions into which sugars are divided. 230. How are sugars graded commercially? 231. What per cent of purity has granulated sugar? 232. How is the coloring material of sugar removed? 233. How is sugar treated to make it whiter? 234. What value as a nutrient does sugar possess? 235. Why should sugar be combined with other nutrients? 236. What foods contain appreciable amounts of sugar? 237. Why is an excessive amount of sugar in a ration undesirable? 238. Does sugar possess more than condimental value? 239. What is the average quantity of sugar consumed in this country? 240. What is maple sugar? 241. How does it differ in composition from other sugar? 242. How is adulterated maple sugar detected? 243. To what extent is granulated sugar adulterated? 244. Why is it not easily adulterated? 245. What are the dextrose sugars? 246. How do they differ chemically from sucrose? 247. What is the inversion of sugar? 248. In what way does acid act upon sugar? 249. How are the acid products removed? 250. What is the food value of glucose? 251. What is molasses? 252. How is it obtained? 253. Of what is it composed? 254. What gives taste and flavor to molasses? 255. How may molasses act upon metalware? 256. What is the food value of molasses? 257. What is sirup? 258. Name three kinds of sirup, and mention materials from which they are prepared. 259. What is the polariscope, and how is it employed in sugar work? 260. What is honey? 261. How does it differ in composition from sugar? 262. How is strained honey adulterated? 263. What materials are used in the preparation of confections? 264. What changes take place in their manufacture? 265. What materials are used for imparting color? 266. What can you say in

regard to the coal tar colors? 267. What should be the position of candy in the dietary? 268. What can you say of the comparative value of cane and beet sugar? 269. How do the commercial grades of sugar compare as to nutritive value? 270. What are some of the impurities in candy? 271. What is saccharine? 272. What are its properties?

CHAPTER VI

LEGUMES AND NUTS

273. What nutrients do the legumes contain in comparatively large amounts? 274. How does the amount of this nutrient compare with that found in meats? 275. Why are legumes valuable crops in general farming and for the feeding of farm animals? 276. Give the general composition of beans. 277. How do beans compare in protein content with cereals? 278. How does the protein of beans differ from that of many other food materials? 279. To what extent are the nutrients of beans digested? 280. What influence does the combination of beans with other foods have upon digestibility? 281. What influence does removal of skins have upon digestibility? 282. In what part of the digestive tract are beans mainly digested? 283. How does the cost of the nutrients in beans compare with that of the nutrients in other foods? 284. How do string beans differ from green beans? 285. Give the general composition, digestibility, and nutritive value of peas. 286. What can you say of the use of copper sulphate in the preparation of canned peas? 287. What nutrients do peanuts contain in large amounts? 288. Give the general composition of nuts. 289. What are the characteristics of pistachio? 290. Give the general composition of the cocoanut. 291. What is cocoanut butter? 292. To what extent may nuts contribute to the nutritive value of a ration?

CHAPTER VII

MILK AND DAIRY PRODUCTS

293. What can you say as to the importance of dairy products in the dietary?

294. Give the general composition of milk. 295. What compound in milk is most variable? 296. To what extent are the nutrients in milk digestible? 297. What influence does milk have upon the digestibility of other foods? 298. Why is cheese cured in cold storage? 299. How can the tendency of a milk diet to produce costiveness be overcome? 300. Why is it necessary to consider the sanitary condition of milk? 301. What factors influence the sanitary condition of milk? 302. What is certified milk? 303. What is pasteurized milk? 304. How can milk be pasteurized for family use? 305. What is tyrotoxicon? 306. What is its source in milk? 307. To what is the color of milk due? 308. To what extent is color associated with fat content? 309. What causes souring of milk? 310. What change occurs in the milk sugar? 311. What are the most favorable conditions for the souring of milk? 312. What are some of the preservatives used in milk. 313. What objection is urged against their use? 314. What is condensed milk? 315. What is buttermilk, and what dietetic value has it? 316. How does goats' milk differ from cows' milk? 317. What is koumiss, and how is it prepared? 318. What are the prepared milks? 319. How does human milk differ in composition from cows' milk? 320. Give the nutritive value of skim milk. 321. What content of fat should cream contain? 322. In what ways is milk adulterated? 323. How are these adulterations detected? 324. Give the general composition of butter. 325. What is the maximum amount of water that a butter may contain without being considered adulterated? 326. What can you say in regard to the digestibility of butter? 327. How is butter adulterated? 328. How does oleomargarine compare in digestibility and food value with butter? 329. What is the food value of butter? 330. How does cheese differ in composition from butter? 331. Give the general composition of cheese. 332. To what are the flavor and odor of cheese due? 333. Why is cheese ripened? 334. What chemical changes take place during ripening? 335. To what extent are the nutrients of cheese digested? 336. Why is cheese sometimes considered indigestible? 337. To what extent do the nutrients of different kinds of cheese vary in digestibility? 338. How does cheese compare in nutritive value and cost with meats? 339. What is cottage cheese? 340. What is Roquefort cheese? 341. Name four kinds of cheese, and say to what each owes its individuality. 342. How is cheese adulterated? 343. Why

are dairy products in older agricultural regions generally cheaper than meats?

CHAPTER VIII

MEATS AND ANIMAL FOOD PRODUCTS

344. Give the general composition of meats. 345. How do meats differ in chemical composition from vegetable foods? 346. What is the principal non-nitrogenous compound of meats, and what of vegetables? 347. Name the different classes of proteins in meats. 348. Which class is present in largest amounts? 349. To what extent are amid compounds present in meats? 350. What characteristics do amids impart to meats? 351. How are alkaloids produced in meats? 352. In what ways does the lean meat of different kinds of animals vary chemically and physically? 353. Give the general composition of beef. 354. What relationship exists between the fat and water content of beef? 355. How much refuse have meats? 356. In what forms are the ash elements (mineral matter) present in meats? 357. How does veal differ in composition from beef? 358. What general changes in composition occur as animals mature? 359. How do these compare with the changes that take place when plants ripen and seeds are produced? 360. How does mutton vary in composition from beef? 361. How does it compare in food value with beef? 362. How do lamb and mutton differ in composition? 363. To what extent do the various cuts differ in composition? 364. How do the more expensive cuts of lamb compare in nutritive value with the less expensive cuts? 365. How does pork differ in composition from other meats? 366. Give the general composition of ham. 367. Give the composition and nutritive value of bacon. 368. How does bacon compare in food value with other meats? 369. How does the character of the fat influence the composition and taste of the meat? 370. What influences the texture or toughness of meats? 371. How do cooked meats compare in composition with raw meats? 372. To what extent are nutrients lost in the boiling of meats? 373. What influence does the temperature of the water in which the meat is placed for cooking have upon the amount of nutrients extracted? 374. To what is the

shrinking of meats in cooking due? 375. Of what does meat extract mainly consist? 376. To what do beef extracts owe their flavor? 377. What is their food value? 378. What is their dietetic value? 379. What is lard? 380. How does it differ in composition from other fats? 381. What is imparted to meats during the smoking process? 382. Why is saltpeter used in the preservation of meats? 383. Do vegetable foods contain nitrates and nitrites? 384. How does poultry resemble and how differ in composition from other meat? 385. Give the characteristics of sound poultry. 386. Give the general composition of fish. 387. How does the flesh of different kinds of fish vary in composition? 388. What influence does salting and preservation have upon composition? 389. How do fish and meat compare in digestibility? 390. How does the mineral matter and phosphate content of fish compare with that of other foods? 391. What are the main nutrients in oysters? 392. Give the general food value of oysters. 393. What is meant by the fattening of oysters? 394. What effect does the character of the water used in fattening have upon the sanitary value? 395. Give the general composition of the egg. 396. How do different parts of the egg differ in composition? 397. How does the egg differ in composition from the potato? 398. Is color an index to the composition of the egg? 399. What effect does cooking have upon the composition of the egg? 400. What factors influence the flavor of eggs? 401. How do different ways of cooking affect the digestibility? 402. Under what conditions can eggs be used economically in the dietary? 403. Why should eggs be purchased and sold by weight? 404. How do canned meats differ in composition from fresh meats? 405. How do the nutrients of canned meats compare in cost with those of fresh meat? 406. What are the advantages of canned meats over fresh meats? 407. What are some of the materials used in the preservation of meats?

CHAPTER IX

CEREALS

408. How are the cereals milled? 409. What are the cereals most commonly used for food purposes? 410. Give the general composition of cereals as a

class. 411. What are the main nutrients in corn preparations? 412. What influence does the more complete removal of the bran and germ of corn have upon its digestibility? 413. How does the cost of nutrients in corn compare with other foods? 414. Why is corn alone not suitable for bread-making purposes? 415. Why should corn be combined in a ration with foods mediumly rich in protein? 416. What change takes place in corn meal from long storage? 417. Give the characteristics and composition of oat preparations. 418. How does removal of the oat hull affect the composition of the product? 419. To what extent do the various oat preparations on the market differ in composition and food value? 420. Do oats contain any special alkaloidal or stimulating principle? 421. Why should oatmeal receive longer and more-thorough cooking than many other foods? 422. To what extent are the nutrients in oatmeal digested? 423. How do wheat preparations differ in general composition from corn and oat preparations? 424. What influence upon the composition of the wheat breakfast foods has partial or complete removal of the bran? 425. What is the effect upon their digestibility and nutritive value? 426. What are the special diabetic flours, and how are they prepared? 427. What are the wheat middlings breakfast foods, and how do they compare in digestibility and food value with bread? 428. How do they differ mechanically? 429. How does barley differ from wheat in general composition? 430. What is barley water, and what nutritive material does it contain? 431. What cereal does rice resemble in composition? 432. With what food materials should rice be combined to make a balanced ration? 433. What can you say as to comparative ease and completeness of digestibility of rice? 434. Why are cereals valuable in the ration? 435. In what way do they take a mechanical part in digestion? 436. What are predigested breakfast foods? 437. How would you determine the general nutritive value of a breakfast food, knowing the kind of cereal from which it was prepared? 438. To what extent are cereals modified or changed in composition by cooking? 439. To what extent are the nutrients of cereal foods digested and absorbed by the body? 440. To what extent do the cereals supply the body with mineral matter? 441. How does the phosphate content of cereals compare with that of meats and milk?

CHAPTER X

WHEAT FLOUR

442. Why is wheat flour especially adapted to bread-making purposes? 443. To what extent may wheat vary in protein content? 444. What are spring wheats? 445. What are winter wheats? 446. Give the general characteristics of each. 447. What are glutinous wheats? 448. What are starchy wheats? 449. Name the different proteids in wheat flour. 450. About how much starch does wheat flour contain? 451. What other carbohydrates are also present? 452. What is the roller process of flour milling? 453. What is meant by the first break? 454. How are the different products of the wheat kernel separated? 455. What is meant by middlings flour? 456. What is break flour? 457. What is patent flour? 458. Name the high grade flours. 459. Name the low grade flours. 460. How are the impurities removed from wheat flour? 461. What per cent of the wheat kernel is returned as flour? As offals? 462. What becomes of the wheat germ during milling? 463. What sized bolting cloths are used in milling? 464. What is graham flour? 465. How does it differ in mechanical and chemical composition from white flour? 466. What is entire wheat flour? 467. How does it differ in physical and chemical composition from white flour? 468. What effect has the refining of flour upon the ash content? 469. How do low and high grade flours differ in chemical composition? 470. How do the wheat offals differ in composition from the flour? 471. What are the factors which influence the composition of flours? 472. What effect does storage have upon the bread-making value of flour? 473. What change takes place when new wheat is stored in an elevator? 474. What is durum wheat flour, and how does it differ from other flour? 475. What gives flour its color? 476. Why is color an index of grade? 477. How is the color of a flour determined? 478. How do flours differ in granulation? 479. How does the granulation affect the physical properties of flour? 480. How is the granulation of flour approximately determined? 481. How is the absorptive capacity of a flour determined? 482. What factors cause a variation in the capacity of flours to absorb water? 483. Give the characteristics of a good gluten. 484. What causes unsound flours? 485.

How is the bread-making value of a flour determined? 486. How are flours bleached? 487. How does bleaching affect the chemical composition of flour? 488. What influence does bleaching have upon bread-making value? 489. Traces of what compounds are formed during bleaching? 490. Are these compounds injurious to health? 491. What effect does bleaching have upon the color of fiber and d 閣 ris particles in flour? 492. Is it possible to bleach low grade flours and cause them to resemble high grade flours? 493. Are flours usually adulterated? 494. Why? 495. How would mineral adulterants be detected? 496. How would the presence of other cereals be detected? 497. How does flour compare in nutritive value with other foods? 498. How does the cost of flour compare with that of other foods? 499. What causes flours to vary so in bread-making value? 500. Why may flours produced from the same type of wheat vary slightly in character from year to year? 501. What relationship exists between the nutritive and bread-making value of a flour?

CHAPTER XI

BREAD AND BREAD MAKING

502. Define leavened and unleavened bread. 503. Why is yeast used in bread making? 504. Give the characteristics of a good loaf of bread. 505. Why is flour used for bread making purposes? 506. Name the eight chemical changes that take place during bread making. 507. To what extent do losses in dry matter occur during bread making? 508. What compounds suffer losses during bread making? 509. What is yeast? 510. What chemical changes does it produce? 511. What becomes of these products during bread making? 512. How is compressed yeast made? 513. What part does the alcohol take in bread making? 514. What temperature is reached in the interior of the loaf during bread making? 515. Through what chemical changes does starch pass during bread making? 516. To what extent are soluble carbohydrates formed? 517. In what way is starch acted upon mechanically? 518. Explain the structure of the starch grains in flour and in dough after they have been acted upon by the yeast ferments. 519. To what extent are acids produced in bread making? 520. What becomes of the acids

formed? 521. How may the acids thus developed affect the properties of other chemical compounds? 522. To what extent are volatile carbon compounds, other than carbon dioxid and alcohol, liberated during bread making? 523. What changes occur to the various proteids during the process of bread making? 524. Why do flours vary in quality of gluten? 525. To what extent do losses of nitrogen occur during bread making? 526. How much of the total nitrogen of flour is present as proteids? 527. How is the fat of flour affected during the process of bread making? 528. What effect does the addition of 10 per cent of wheat starch to flour have upon the size of the loaf? 529. What effect does the addition of 10 per cent of wheat gluten to flour have upon the size of the loaf? 530. What relationship exists between gluten content and capacity of a flour to absorb water? 531. Give the general composition of bread. 532. What factors influence its composition? 533. What effect does the use of skim milk and lard in bread making have upon composition? 534. How does the temperature of the flour influence the bread-making process? 535. Why is it necessary to vary the process of bread making in order to get the best results with different kinds of flour? 536. To what extent are the nutrients of bread digested? 537. How does graham bread compare in digestibility with white bread? 538. How do graham and entire wheat breads compare in nutritive value with white bread? 539. What value do graham and entire wheat breads have in the dietary? 540. Why is white bread generally preferable in the dietary of the laboring man? 541. How do graham and entire wheat flours compare in chemical composition with white flour? 542. How do they compare in mechanical composition? 543. To what is the difference in digestibility supposed to be due? 544. Are graham and entire wheat breads necessary in a ration as a source of mineral elements? 545. What is the main difference in composition between old and new bread? 546. How do different kinds of bread made from the same flour compare in composition and nutritive value? 447. How does toast differ in composition from bread? 548. What influence does toasting have upon digestibility? 549. What is gained by toasting bread? 550. How does bread compare in nutritive value with other cereal foods? 551. How does bread compare in nutritive value with animal foods?

CHAPTER XII

BAKING POWDERS

552. What is a baking powder? 553. What are the two kinds of materials which baking powders contain? 554. Name the different types of baking powders. 555. How does baking powder differ in its action from yeast? 556. What are the cream of tartar baking powders? 557. What is the nature of the residue which they leave? 558. What are the phosphate baking powders? 559. What is the nature of the residue which they leave? 560. Why is the mineral phosphate not considered equally valuable with that naturally present in foods? 561. What are the alum baking powders? 562. What residue is left from the alum powders? 563. Which of the three classes of baking powders is considered the least objectionable? 564. Why is a new baking powder preferable to one that has been kept a long time? 565. Why should baking powders be kept in tin cans, and not in paper? 566. Why are fillers used in the manufacture of baking powders? 567. How may a baking powder be prepared at home? 568. How does such a baking powder compare in cost and efficiency with those purchased in the market?

CHAPTER XIII

VINEGARS, SPICES, AND CONDIMENTS

569. What is vinegar? 570. How is it made? 571. Give the three chemical changes that take place in its preparation. 572. Why is air necessary in the last stage of the process? 573. What ferments take part in the production of vinegar? 574. What is malt vinegar? 575. What materials other than apples can be used in the preparation of vinegar? 576. Give the characteristics of a good vinegar. 577. In what ways are vinegars adulterated? 578. What food value has vinegar? 579. Why should vinegars not be stored in metalware? 580. What dietetic value has vinegar? 581. To what materials do the spices owe their value? 582. What is pepper? 583. What is the difference between white and black pepper? 584. What compounds give pepper its

characteristics? 585. How are peppers adulterated? 586. What is mustard? 587. Give its general composition. 588. How is it adulterated? 589. What is ginger? 590. How is it prepared for the market? 591. Give its general composition. 592. What is cinnamon? 593. What is cassia? 594. What gives these their taste and flavor? 595. What are cloves? 596. How are they prepared? 597. What is mace? 598. What is nutmeg? 599. Do the spices have any food value? 600. What is their dietetic value? 601. Why is excessive use of some of the spices objectionable?

CHAPTER XIV

TEA, COFFEE, CHOCOLATE, AND COCOA

602. What is tea? Name the two plants from which it is obtained, the countries where each grows best, and the number of flushes each yields. 603. Upon what does the quality and grade of tea depend? 604. Give differences in the preparation and composition of green and black teas. 605. The characteristic flavor of tea is imparted by what compound? 606. To what compound are its peculiar physiological properties due? 607. What can you say of the protein in tea as to amount and food value? 608. Why should tea--especially green tea--be infused for a very short time, never boiled? 609. What effect has tannin upon the digestion of proteids? 610. What three points are considered in judging a tea? 611. What is the most common form of tea adulteration? 612. Describe the coffee plant and fruit, and its method of preparation for market. 613. What is the difference in the chemical composition of tea and coffee? 614. Name the characteristic alkaloid of coffee. How does it compare with theme? 615. Why may coffee not be considered a food? 616. Tell different ways in which coffee may be adulterated. 617. Which is more commonly practiced, tea or coffee adulteration? Why? 618. How may real coffee be distinguished from chicory? Why? 619. Name the three kinds of coffee in general use. Give distinguishing features of each. Which is usually considered best? 620. From what are cocoa and chocolate obtained? 621. Give the two methods of preparing cocoa. 622. What alkaloid similar to the theme and caffeine of tea

and coffee is present in cocoa and chocolate? 623. What is the difference in preparation of cocoa and chocolate? 624. What are cereal coffee-substitutes? 625. What nutritive value have they? 626. How do they differ in composition from coffee? 627. To what extent does cocoa add to the nutritive value of a ration? 628. What is plain chocolate? 629. Why do chocolate preparations vary so widely in composition? 630. What treatment is given to the cocoa bean in its preparation for commerce? 631. What treatment is sometimes given to prevent separation of the cocoa fat? 632. In what ways may cocoa and chocolate preparations be adulterated?

CHAPTER XV

DIGESTIBILITY OF FOODS

633. Define the term nutrient. 634. Do all the nutrients of food have the same degree of digestibility? 635. What is a digestion coefficient? 636. How is the digestibility of a food determined? 637. What volatile products are formed during the digestion of food? 638. Define digestible protein; digestible carbohydrates, digestible fat. 639. What is the available energy of a ration? 640. How is it determined? 641. How do the nutrients, protein, fat, and carbohydrates, compare as to available energy? 642. Why is it necessary to consider the caloric value of a ration? 643. Is the protein molecule as completely oxidized in the body as starch or fat? 644. What residue is left from the digestion of protein? 645. What part do the soluble ferments take in digestion? 646. To what extent are the nutrients of animal foods digested? 647. Which nutrient, protein or fat, is the most completely digested? 648. How do vegetable foods compare in digestibility with animal foods? 649. What effect does cellulose have upon digestibility? 650. Which of the nutrients of vegetables, protein or carbohydrates, is more completely digested? 651. What mechanical value may cellulose have in a ration? 652. Why must bulk be considered in a ration, as well as nutrient content? 653. Name the eight most important factors influencing the digestibility of foods. 654. To what extent does the combination of foods affect the digestibility of the nutrients? 655. Why does a mixed ration give better results than when

only a single food is used? 656. How does the amount consumed affect the completeness of the digestive process? 657. To what extent does the method of preparing food affect digestibility? 658. What is gained, so far as digestibility is concerned, by the cooking of foods? 659. To what extent does the mechanical condition of food affect its digestibility? 660. Why is it desirable to have some coarsely granulated foods in a ration? 661. Why should the ration not be composed exclusively of finely granulated foods? 662. Why is some coarsely granulated food more essential in the dietary of the sedentary than in the dietary of the laborer? 663. How does palatability affect the digestive process? 664. Do psychological processes in any way affect digestion? 665. What physiological properties do some foods possess? 666. To what are these physiological properties due? 667. To what extent is individuality a factor in digestion? 668. To what extent does digestibility differ with individuals? 669. Why do some foods affect individuals in different ways? 670. Why is it necessary that the quantity, quality, and character of the food should vary with different individuals? 671. In what different ways is the expression "digestibility of a food" used? 672. Why is it necessary to consider the digestibility of food, as well as its composition? 673. Does the digestibility of a food necessarily indicate the economic uses that will be made of it by the body? 674. How is it possible for one food containing 10 per cent of digestible protein, and other nutrients in like amounts, to be more valuable than another food with the same per cent of digestible protein and other nutrients? 675. How is it possible for one food to contain less total protein than another food and yet be more valuable from a nutritive point of view? 676. Why is it necessary to consider the mechanical condition of a food and its combination with other foods, as well as its chemical composition? 677. What effect does lack of a good supply of air have upon the completeness of the digestion process? 678. In what ways does the digestion of food resemble the combustion of fuel? 679. What is gained by a study of the digestibility of foods? 680. Why may two foods of the same general character give different results when used for nutritive purposes?

CHAPTER XVI

COMPARATIVE COST AND VALUE OF FOODS

681. To what extent do the nutritive value and the market price of foods vary? 682. How is the value of one food expressed in terms of another food? 683. How determine the amount of nutrients that can be procured in a food for a given sum of money? 684. How compare the amounts of nutrients that can be procured in two foods for a given sum of money? 685. How is it possible to determine approximately which of two foods is cheaper, when the price and composition of the foods are known? 686. To what nutrient is preference usually given in assigning a value to a food? 687. When the difference in this nutrient between two foods is small, then the preference is given to what nutrients? 688. At ordinary prices, what are the cheapest vegetable foods? 689. What are among the cheapest animal foods? 690. Why is it not possible to determine the value of a food absolutely from its composition and digestibility? 691. Why is it necessary to consider the physical as well as the chemical composition of foods? 692. What proportion of the income of the laboring man is usually expended for food? 693. What are the most expensive foods? 694. What foods furnish the largest amount of nutrients at the least cost?

CHAPTER XVII

DIETARY STUDIES

695. What is a dietary study? 696. How is a dietary study made? 697. What is the value of the dietary study of a family? 698. To what extent does the protein in the dietary range? 699. Why is a scant amount of protein in a ration undesirable? 700. Why is an excess of protein in the ration undesirable? 701. What are dietary standards? 702. How are such standards obtained? 703. Why is it desirable in a ration to secure the protein and other nutrients from a variety rather than from a few foods? 704. Why is it necessary to consider the caloric value of a ration? 705. How is this determined? 706. What is a wide nutritive ratio? 707. What is a narrow

nutritive ratio? 708. Why should the amount of nutrients consumed vary with the work performed? 709. How should the nutrients be apportioned among the meals? 710. What are some of the most common dietary errors? 711. What analogy exists between human and animal feeding? 712. What is gained by the rational feeding of both humans and animals? 713. What use can be made of the results of dietary studies for improvement of the dietary? 714. Why is it not possible for animal foods to compete in economy with cereal and vegetable foods? 715. Is a well-balanced ration and one containing an ample supply of nutrients necessarily an expensive ration? 716. Show how it is possible for one family to spend less money for food than another family, and yet secure more digestible nutrients and energy. 717. What are some of the most erroneous ideas as to food values? 718. Why is it necessary to consider previously acquired food habits in the selection of foods? 719. In general, what portion of the nutrients of a ration should be derived from vegetable foods, and what portion from meats? 720. To what extent may a ration vary from the dietary standards? 721. Why are some inexpensive foods often expensive when prepared for the table? 722. What are some of the ways in which the cost of a ration can be decreased without sacrificing nutritive value? 723. Why do different nationalities acquire distinct food habits? 724. Why is it not possible to make sudden and radical changes in the dietary? 725. Why is it not possible for a dietary which gives ample satisfaction for one class of people to be applied to another class with equal satisfaction? 726. What relationship exists between the dietary of a nation and its physical development? 727. What relationship exists between dietary habits and mental development and vigor? 728. Why is it unnecessary and undesirable to regulate absolutely the amount of nutrients consumed in the daily ration? 729. What is the general tendency as to quantity of food and amount of nutrients consumed? 730. Why do people of sedentary habits require a different dietary from those pursuing active, out-of-door occupations?

CHAPTER XVIII

RATIONAL FEEDING OF MAN

731. What is the object of the rational feeding of man? 732. On what is it based? 733. How does it compare with the rational feeding of animals? 734. What is a standard ration? 735. How is it determined? 736. To what extent may the nutrients of a ration vary from the standard? 737. How do you combine foods to form a balanced ration? 738. What foods are valuable for supplying protein? 739. What foods supply fats? 740. What foods are rich in carbohydrates? 741. What other requisites should a ration have in addition to supplying the necessary nutrients? 742. Why is it necessary to consider the calorie value of a ration? 743. If a ration contained an excess of carbohydrates and a scant amount of protein, how could it be improved? 744. How do you calculate the nutrients in a fraction of a pound of food? 745. Give the amounts of the common food materials, as potatoes, bread, butter, milk, and cheese, ordinarily combined to form a ration. 746. To what extent may foods differ in composition from the average analysis given? 747. What foods are subject to the greatest and what foods to the least variation?

CHAPTER XIX

WATER

748. Why is water regarded as a food? 749. Does it enter chemically into the composition of plants? Of animals? 750. In addition to serving as a food, why is water necessary for life processes? 751. In what ways may water be improved? 752. What are the most common forms of impurities? 753. What are the mineral impurities of water? 754. What is their source? 755. What effect do some of these minerals have upon the value of the water? 756. What causes some waters to dissolve limestone? 757. What are permanently hard waters? 758. To what is temporary hardness in water due? 759. What is the best way to remove mineral matter from water? 760. What are the organic impurities of water? 761. What are the sources of the organic impurities? 762. What change does the organic matter of water undergo? 763. What becomes of the nitrogen of the organic matter? 764. What does the presence of nitrates in water indicate? Nitrites? 765. What is the total

solid matter of a water, and how is it obtained? 766. Define the terms free ammonia; albuminoid ammonia. 767. What does the presence of chlorine in a surface well water indicate? 768. Explain natural purification of water. 769. Can natural purification always be relied upon? 770. Why does the character of the drinking water affect health? 771. What diseases are mainly caused by impure drinking water? 772. With what materials in water are the disease-producing organisms associated? 773. Why should a water of questionable purity be boiled? 774. State how the boiling should be done, to be effective. 775. Why should boiled water receive further care in its storage? 776. What effect does improvement of the water supply of a city have upon the death rate? 777. How may connections between cesspools and surface well waters be traced? 778. What impurities do rain waters contain? 779. Explain the workings of the Pasteur and Berkefeld water filters. 780. Why must special attention be given to cleaning the water filter? 781. Explain the processes employed for the removal of mechanical impurities of water by sedimentation and the use of chemicals. 782. Why should such purification be under the supervision of a chemist or bacteriologist? 783. What effect does freezing have upon the purity of water? 784. Why are precautions necessary in the use of ice for refrigeration? 785. What are mineral waters? 786. How are artificial mineral waters prepared? 787. What are the more common materials used in their preparation? 788. Why should mineral waters be extensively used only by the advice of a physician? 789. What are some of the materials used for softening water? 790. Which are the least objectionable of these materials? 791. Which are the most objectionable? 792. What can you say of the use of ammonia and ammonium carbonate for softening waters? 793. In washing clothing after contagious diseases, what materials may be used for disinfecting? 794. Why, in softening waters for household purposes, must caustic soda, potash, and bleaching powder be used with caution? 795. Why is it necessary to determine by trial the material most suitable for softening water? 796. What advantage, from a pecuniary point of view, results from the improvement of the water supply of a community?

CHAPTER XX

FOOD IN ITS RELATION TO HOUSEHOLD SANITATION AND STORAGE

797. What are the compounds usually determined in a food analysis? 798. Does such an analysis necessarily indicate the presence of injurious compounds? 799. What are the sources of the injurious organic compounds in foods? 800. Why is it necessary to consider sanitary condition as well as chemical composition? 801. What are the sources of contamination of foods? 802. What is the object of the sanitary inspection of food? 803. How may flies carry germ diseases? 804. Why should food be protected from impure air and dust particles? 805. Why should places where vegetables are stored be well ventilated? 806. How may the dirt adhering to vegetables be the carrier of germ diseases? 807. Why should the cellar in which food is stored be in a sanitary condition? 808. What effect does the cleaning of streets and improvement of the sanitation of cities have upon the death rate? 809. Name the three natural disinfectants, and explain the action of each. 810. Why must dishes and utensils in which foods are placed be thoroughly cleaned? 811. Explain the principle of refrigeration. 812. What kind of ferment action may take place at a low temperature? 813. Why is some ventilation necessary in refrigeration? 814. What effect does refrigeration have upon the composition of food? 815. What relationship exists between unsanitary condition of soils about dwellings and contamination of the food? 816. Why should special attention be given to the sanitary disposal of kitchen refuse? 817. Name the ways in which this can be accomplished. 818. How may foods become contaminated through imperfect plumbing? 819. Mention the conditions necessary in order to keep foods sanitary.

###